Veterinary Nursing
Self-Assessment Questions and Answers

3rd edition

For Butterworth-Heinemann:

Commissioning Editor: Mary Seager
Development Editor: Catharine Steers
Project Manager: Derek Robertson
Designer: Andy Chapman

Veterinary Nursing:

Self-Assessment Questions and Answers

Third edition

J E Ouston MA VetMB MRCVS
Veterinary Surgeon and Lecturer in Veterinary Nursing
MYF Training, Aldershot

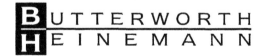

EDINBURGH LONDON NEW YORK OXFORD
PHILADELPHIA ST LOUIS SYDNEY TORONTO 2004

BUTTERWORTH-HEINEMANN
An imprint of Elsevier Limited

First published 1997

ISBN 07506 8781 9

British Library Cataloguing in Publication Data
A catalogue record for this book is available from the British Library

Library of Congress Cataloguing in Publication Data
A catalog record for this book is available from the Library of Congress

Notice
Veterinary knowledge is constantly changing. Standard safety precautions must be
followed, but as new research and clinical experience broaden our knowledge,
changes in treatment and drug therapy may become necessary or appropriate. Readers
are advised to check the most current product information provided by the
manufacturer of each drug to be administered to verify the recommended dose, the
method and duration of administration, and contraindications. It is the responsibility
of the practitioner, relying on experience and knowledge of the patient, to determine
dosages and the best treatment for each individual patient. Neither the Publisher nor
the author assumes any liability for any injury and/or damage to persons or property
arising from this publication.

Transferred to Digital Printing 2010

 your source for books,
journals and multimedia
in the health sciences
www.elsevierhealth.com

Contents

Preface

I wrote my first set of multiple choice books in 1996, and these proved to be very popular with student veterinary nurses, especially as a means of testing themselves prior to the Royal College of Veterinary Surgeons' examinations. In 1998 the syllabus was changed, and NVQs were introduced. At this stage the books were updated into a single volume, and the changes in the syllabus incorporated. Now it is time for a third edition to complement the standard nursing text, *Veterinary Nursing*, which has been completely rewritten. The book contains a completely new set of questions, and I hope that a new generation of student veterinary nurses will get as much out of the book as previous students have told me they did.

The book includes both NVQ level 2 and NVQ level 3 questions, and has been compiled to follow the chapter layout of *Veterinary Nursing* (3rd edition), edited by Lane & Cooper. However, I have not included questions on behaviour problems or bereavement, since these are not subjects on which students will be examined by the RCVS. At the beginning of each subject I have given the number of questions, to provide an indication of the amount of time that should be allowed. In the RCVS examinations, each paper consists of 90 questions and students have 90 minutes in which to complete it. Therefore, to practise examination technique, one minute should be allowed for each question. Each question is presented with four possible answers, from which the one correct answer has to be selected.

When answering multiple choice questions, there are a few general tips that should be followed:

- Always read the question or opening statement carefully, checking for words like 'not', or 'untrue'. It is easy to lose marks simply by not reading the questions properly.
- If there are calculations in the section being covered, it may be best to do the other questions first and come back to the calculations. For many people they take longer than one minute, but they carry no more marks than any other question, so it is important that not too much time is spent

on these such that there is not enough time for the rest of the paper.

- It is also important not to rush the questions. Although it may seem that time will be a problem, one minute per question is actually plenty, and most students easily finish within the allocated time. Therefore, take time to read the questions fully, and make sure that every question has an answer.

The answers for all the questions can be found in a separate section at the end of the book. I have given full explanations for the answers, and I hope that this book will not only act as a means of self assessment, but also help students to understand the subjects more fully.

JEO

Questions

1 Anatomy and physiology

149 Questions

Terminology and directional terms

1. **Which term relates to structures closer to the trunk?**

   A Cranial
   B Ventral
   C Medial
   D Proximal

2. **The under surface of the hind paw is described as**

   A Ventral
   B Caudal
   C Palmar
   D Plantar

3. **Which is the most rostral structure?**

   A Ear
   B Tail
   C Zygomatic arch
   D Foramen magnum

Body fluid compartments

4. **Salt is an electrolyte which dissolves into ions in water. Which anion is found in common salt?**

    A Sodium
    B Potassium
    C Chloride
    D Carbonate

5. **What proportion of the total body water is found within cells?**

    A 20%
    B 66%
    C 33%
    D 70%

6. **The regulation of pH within the body is carried out by all the following except:**

    A Kidneys
    B Lungs
    C Heart
    D Plasma

7. **The pH scale provides a measure of the acidity of a solution. Which of the following solutions is the most acidic?**

    A A solution with pH 7.0
    B A solution with pH 5.5
    C A solution with pH 13.0
    D A solution with pH 8.0

8. **How much fluid does an average animal lose per day through respiration?**

    A 5 ml/kg/24hours
    B 10 ml/kg/24hours
    C 15 ml/kg/24 hours
    D 20 ml/kg/24 hours

9. **A solution which exerts a higher osmotic pressure than body fluids is**

   A Isotonic
   B Hypertonic
   C Hypotonic
   D Hyperbaric

10. **Which statement is true about the constituents of intracellular fluid?**

    A The main cation is sodium
    B Bicarbonate and chloride are the main anions
    C There is usually very little protein present
    D Phosphate is the main anion

Cell structure

11. **Adenosine triphosphate (ATP) is formed within cells by which of the following organelles?**

    A Ribosomes
    B Vacuoles
    C Mitochondria
    D Centrioles

12. **There are four stages in mitosis. Which is the correct sequence?**

    A Prophase, metaphase, anaphase, telophase
    B Metaphase, telophase, anaphase, prophase
    C Anaphase, telophase, metaphase, prophase
    D Prophase, telophase, metaphase, anaphase

13. **Which term is used to describe the way in which some cells are able to engulf solid particles?**

    A Phagocytosis
    B Exocytosis
    C Endocytosis
    D Pinocytosis

14. **Which organelle is responsible for transport of materials around the cell?**

    A Golgi apparatus
    B Ribosomes
    C Endoplasmic reticulum
    D Lysosomes

15. **The cell cycle consists of a number of stages. What takes place during interphase?**

    A The nuclear membrane breaks down at the start of cell division
    B The cell rests between cell divisions
    C The daughter cells reform their nuclear membranes
    D The chromatids separate from each other along the mitotic spindle

Basic tissue types

16. **Which of the following is an example of a dense connective tissue?**

    A Tendon
    B Adipose tissue
    C Cartilage
    D Bone

17. **Which of the following best describes areolar tissue?**

    A It contains large numbers of fat cells, and is used as an energy store
    B It is found surrounding muscle fibres, and forms the muscle sheath
    C It is found surrounding nerve cells, and improves impulse conduction
    D It is found beneath skin, and is used as a packing material

18. **The type of epithelium found lining blood vessels is**

    A Simple squamous epithelium
    B Stratified squamous epithelium
    C Simple cuboidal epithelium
    D Transitional epithelium

19. **Intervertebral discs are found between the centra of adjacent vertebrae and consist of which form of cartilage?**

    A Hyaline cartilage
    B Fibrocartilage
    C Elastic cartilage
    D None of the above

The body cavities

20. The pleura lining the inside the ribcage is called

A Diaphragmatic pleura
B Pulmonary pleura
C Costal pleura
D Visceral pleura

21. Which organ is retroperitoneal?

A Liver
B Stomach
C Kidney
D Bladder

22. The structure found in the mediastinum is the

A Azygous vein
B Thyroid gland
C Prostate gland
D Spleen

23. Which of the following best defines the term mesentery?

A The space between the right and left pleural cavities
B The peritoneal fold lying between the abdominal wall and the stomach
C The peritoneal fold lying between the abdominal wall and the intestine .
D The fold of peritoneum between the uterus and the abdominal wall

The skeletal system

24. **There are several cell types associated with the skeletal system. All of the following can be found there except:**

    A Osteoblasts
    B Osteoclasts
    C Mast cells
    D Chondrocytes

25. **The bones that form by intramembranous ossification are**

    A Sesamoid bones
    B Splanchnic bones
    C Long bones
    D Flat bones

26. **The part of a long bone known as the diaphysis is**

    A The end of the bone
    B The growth plate of the bone
    C The shaft of the bone
    D The cavity within the centre of the bone

27. **Which of the following is an example of a flat bone?**

    A Parietal bone
    B Atlas
    C Tibia
    D Patella

28. **The skeleton is divided into the axial and appendicular skeleton. Which bone does not form part of the axial skeleton?**

    A Maxilla
    B Pubis
    C Manubrium
    D Rib

29. **The splanchnic skeleton includes which of the following bones?**

    A Fabella
    B Frontal bone
    C Femur
    D Os penis

30. **The cranium is the bony box that contains the brain. Which skull bone forms the floor of the cranium?**

    A Frontal bone
    B Temporal bone
    C Sphenoid bone
    D Occipital bone

31. **Which of the following bones contains a sinus?**

    A Mandible
    B Maxilla
    C Parietal bone
    D Temporal bone

32. **Which of the following statements about vertebrae is correct?**

    A There are 5 cervical vertebrae
    B The 3 sacral vertebrae are separate in the cat
    C The coccygeal vertebrae are different to the caudal vertebrae
    D The largest vertebrae in the spine are the 7 lumbar vertebrae

33. **The long thin skull of an animal such as a Borzoi can be described as**

    A Doliocephalic
    B Mesocephalic
    C Brachycephalic
    D Mesaticephalic

34. Fovea are found on which vertebrae?

A Coccygeal
B Thoracic
C Lumbar
D Cervical

35. The fabellae are located

A Adjacent to the elbow
B Adjacent to the hock
C Adjacent to the carpus
D Adjacent to the stifle

36. The large bone that forms the point of the hock is called the

A Calcaneus
B Talus
C Accessory tarsal bone
D Tibial tarsal bone

37. Which term describes the movement in which the angle between two bones forming a joint is reduced?

A Flexion
B Extension
C Protraction
D Adduction

38. The greater trochanter is found on which of the following bones?

A Humerus
B Tibia
C Femur
D Radius

39. The type of joint that allows the most movement is a

A Diarthrosis
B Synarthrosis
C Amphiarthrosis
D Symphysis

The muscular system

40. **The type of muscle also described as striated muscle is**

A Smooth muscle
B Skeletal muscle
C Cardiac muscle
D Visceral muscle

41. **A motor unit is defined as**

A The unit of muscle contraction
B The fibres within a muscle cell that slide over each other
C A bundle of muscles within one region of a limb
D A group of muscle cells supplied by one nerve fibre

42. **The prime protractor of the forelimb is**

A Biceps femoris
B Brachialis
C Biceps brachii
D Brachiocephalicus

43. **Which of the following muscles is an extrinsic muscle of the forelimb?**

A Trapezius
B Brachialis
C Biceps brachii
D Infraspinatus

44. **The muscle never involved in respiration is**

A Latissimus dorsi
B External intercostals
C External abdominal oblique
D Transversus abdominis

45. Extension of the elbow is caused by which of the following muscles?

A Brachialis
B Biceps brachii
C Supraspinatus
D Triceps brachii

46. Which muscle has its origin on the spinous processes of the thoracic vertebrae?

A Latissimus dorsi
B Pectineus
C Infraspinatus
D Semimembranosus

47. The Achilles tendon is made up of the tendons of insertion of four muscles. The tendon of which of the following does not form part of this structure?

A Gastrocnemius
B Anterior tibial
C Semitendinosus
D Biceps femoris

48. Which statement is true about muscle contraction?

A There needs to be a supply of free sodium ions within the cell for contraction to occur
B There are filaments within the muscle cells which slide over each other
C The filaments in the cells are made of collagen
D A muscle contraction can be called a sarcomere

49. Of the four abdominal muscles, which has its insertion on the pelvis via the prepubic tendon?

A Transversus abdominis
B External abdominal oblique
C Internal abdominal oblique
D Rectus abdominis

50. Gastrocnemius is best described as a

    A Hip flexor and stifle extensor
    B Stifle flexor and hock extensor
    C Hip extensor and stifle flexor
    D Stifle extensor and hock flexor

The nervous system

51. Which statement is true about neuron structure?

A Every neuron has at least one axon and one dendron
B Dendrites carry impulses away from the cell body
C A neuron has only one axon
D The axons of all neurons are myelinated

52. A synapse is found in which of the following sites?

A In the central canal of the spinal cord
B Within a neuron
C Between two neurons
D In the dorsal root ganglion

53. The true statement about the function of the parasympathetic nervous system is that

A It stimulates salivation
B It causes piloerection
C It causes pupil dilation
D It speeds up the heart rate

54. The central nervous system (CNS) develops from which tissue layer within the embryo?

A The ectoderm layer of the inner cell mass
B The mesoderm layer of the inner cell mass
C The endoderm layer
D The trophoblast

55. The part of the brain responsible for conscious thought is

A The cerebrum
B The hypothalamus
C The cerebellum
D The medulla oblongata

56. **Where is the cerebral aqueduct found within the central nervous system?**

    A Forebrain
    B Midbrain
    C Hindbrain
    D Spinal cord

57. **The sensory receptors found in skin are**

    A Proprioceptors
    B Chemoreceptors
    C Baroreceptors
    D Nociceptors

58. **Which of the following cranial nerves carries parasympathetic neurons to the head?**

    A Oculomotor, cranial nerve III
    B Trochlear, cranial nerve IV
    C Vestibulo-cochlear, cranial nerve VIII
    D Vagus, cranial nerve X

59. **The cranial nerve that conveys the sense of hearing is the**

    A Auditory nerve
    B Vagus nerve
    C Vestibulo-cochlear nerve
    D Cerebellar nerve

60. **Sympathetic neurons leave the central nervous system with which nerves?**

    A Cranial and sacral nerves
    B Cervical and thoracic nerves
    C Thoracic and lumbar nerves
    D Lumbar and sacral nerves

61. **The term plexus can be used to describe**

    A A nerve
    B A blood vessel
    C A network
    D A muscle

62. The parasympathetic nervous system uses which of the following neurotransmitters?

A Dopamine
B Acetyl choline
C Adrenaline
D Noradrenaline

63. Which of the following is a sensory neuron?

A Afferent somatic neuron
B Efferent autonomic neuron
C Intercalated neuron
D Efferent somatic neuron

64. Gustation is another word for

A Smell
B Taste
C Swallowing
D Digestion

65. Where in the eye is the limbus located?

A It is the junction between the sclera and the cornea
B It is the point where the conjunctiva folds back on itself, where the lacrimal gland opens
C It is the point at which upper and lower eyelid meet
D It is the name given to the edge of the tapetum lucidum

66. How does an animal focus light onto the retina?

A By changing the size of the pupil through the use of smooth muscles in the iris
B By altering the pull on the lens via the suspensory ligament and ciliary body
C By altering the curvature of the cornea
D By altering the density of the aqueous humour in the anterior chamber of the eye

67. **The uvea (uveal tract) consists of all of the following except the**

    A Choroid
    B Iris
    C Ciliary body
    D Pupil

68. **Which of the following is a conditional reflex?**

    A The jerk of the stifle in response to the tendon of quadriceps femoris being tapped with a small hammer
    B The twitch of the panniculus muscle in response to a pin-prick
    C Salivation at the sight of the fridge being opened
    D The withdrawal of the foot if the web between the toes is pinched

69. **The function of the ossicles is to**

    A Transmit sound waves across the middle ear cavity
    B Determine the position of the head relative to the earth
    C Detect head movement
    D Equalise the air pressure between the middle ear and the environment

70. **The structures that make up the vestibular apparatus in the ear are**

    A The external ear canal and pinna
    B The utricle and saccule (the otolith organs) and the semicircular canals
    C The organ of Corti and the ossicles
    D The eustachian tube and the ossicles

The endocrine system

71. **The chorion secretes the hormone chorionic gonadotrophin. What is its function?**

    A To maintain the corpus luteum
    B To provide feedback to the pituitary and prevent the release of follicle stimulating hormone and luteinising hormone
    C To encourage the production of prostaglandins needed to start parturition
    D To bring the animal back into season

72. **The anterior pituitary secretes which of the following hormones?**

    A Aldosterone
    B Adrenocorticotrophic hormone
    C Oestrogen
    D Parathyroid hormone

73. **Which of the following does not contain endocrine tissue?**

    A Mammary gland
    B Kidney
    C Small intestine
    D Pancreas

74. **Addison's disease is the result of which of the following hormone imbalances?**

    A Lack of anti-diuretic hormone (ADH)
    B Excessive amounts of glucocorticoids
    C Lack of growth hormone
    D Lack of mineralocorticoids

75. **The hormone that regulates metabolic rate is**

    A Parathyroid hormone
    B Thyrocalcitonin
    C Growth hormone
    D Thyroxine

76. Where is oxytocin produced?

A Anterior pituitary
B Ovary
C Posterior pituitary
D Placenta

77. The function of interstitial cell stimulating hormone is to

A Stimulate the release of testosterone from the cells of Leydig in the testis
B Stimulate the intermediary cells in the pancreas to secrete somatostatin
C Stimulate the development of the follicles within the ovary
D Stimulate cells in the kidney to reabsorb sodium

78. When calcium levels in the bloodstream rise above normal, which hormone is normally released?

A Parathyroid hormone
B Thyroxine
C Thyrocalcitonin
D Glucagon

The blood vascular system

79. **The bloodstream carries out all of the following functions except**

    A To carry oxygen and carbon dioxide to and from the tissues
    B To remove excess interstitial fluid from the spaces between cells and prevent the formation of oedema
    C To carry heat around the body
    D To protect the animal from disease

80. **The pH of blood is**

    A 6.5
    B 7.0
    C 7.4
    D 8.5

81. **Of the following cells found in blood, which is the smallest?**

    A Erythrocyte
    B Neutrophil
    C Monocyte
    D Lymphocyte

82. **Where is the hormone erythropoietin produced?**

    A Liver
    B Kidney
    C Heart
    D Bone marrow

83. **Which white blood cell has granules in its cytoplasm containing histamine?**

    A Basophil
    B Lymphocyte
    C Eosinophil
    D Monocyte

84. **The white blood cells responsible for the production of antibodies are**

    A B-lymphocytes
    B Monocytes
    C Neutrophils
    D T-lymphocytes

85. **In which cells would you see Howell-Jolly bodies?**

    A Erythrocytes
    B Basophils
    C Thrombocytes
    D Reticulocytes

86. **Which of the following tissue layers of the heart is a serous membrane?**

    A Endocardium
    B Myocardium
    C Epicardium
    D Chordae tendineae

87. **The bicuspid valve can also be called the**

    A Tricuspid valve
    B Mitral valve
    C Aortic valve
    D Pulmonic valve

88. **The true statement about the blood flow through the heart is**

    A Deoxygenated blood returns to the heart from the body via the vena cava
    B Oxygenated blood returns to the heart from the lungs via the pulmonary artery
    C Deoxygenated blood passes through the left side of the heart
    D Deoxygenated blood leaves the heart via the aorta

89. What are Purkinje fibres?

A Groups of heart cells involved with starting the wave of contraction in the atria

B The means of electrical connection between adjacent heart muscle cells

C Specialised conducting cells which spread the wave of contraction through the walls of the ventricles

D The fibres which connect the valve leaflets to the walls of the ventricles, preventing the valves being turned inside out

90. The first heart sound, the lubb, is the sound of which valves closing?

A The aortic and pulmonic valves

B The tricuspid and aortic valves

C The semilunar valves

D The atrio-ventricular valves

91. Which artery carries blood to the stomach, spleen and liver?

A Coronary artery

B Coeliac artery

C Cranial mesenteric artery

D Subclavian artery

92. The statement/s true of both veins and lymph vessels is/are

A The vessels contain valves to ensure one way flow

B The fluid within the vessels is deoxygenated

C Skeletal muscle contractions help move the fluid

D All the above are true

93. The hepatic portal vein connects which two structures in the circulation?

A The vena cava and the liver

B The capillary network of the intestines and the liver

C The thoracic duct and the cranial vena cava

D The liver and the azygous vein

94. Which of the following lymph nodes can you not normally palpate?

   A   Axillary
   B   Submandibular
   C   Popliteal
   D   Retropharyngeal

95. Both lymphoid and myeloid tissue are found in the

   A   Bone marrow
   B   Spleen
   C   Lymph nodes
   D   Thymus

The respiratory system

96. **In which sequence does air pass through the structures of the respiratory system on its way to the lungs?**

    A Nares, pharynx, larynx, trachea, bronchi, bronchioles
    B Nares, larynx, pharynx, trachea, bronchioles, bronchi
    C Nares, pharynx, larynx, trachea, bronchioles, bronchi
    D Nares, larynx, pharynx, bronchi, trachea, bronchioles

97. **Vocal sounds are produced in which region of the respiratory tract?**

    A Trachea
    B Pharynx
    C Larynx
    D Nasal chambers

98. **The opening to the larynx is the**

    A Epiglottis
    B Glottis
    C Hyoid
    D Pharynx

99. **Which statement is true about the lungs?**

    A Both left and right lungs have the same number of lobes
    B The left lung has 4 lobes, and the right has 3
    C The caudal lobe can also be called the cardiac lobe
    D The right lung has an accessory lobe

100. **The term 'dead space' refers to**

    A The parts of the respiratory tract above the level of the trachea
    B The areas of the lungs rarely used for respiration except in laboured breathing
    C The parts of the respiratory tract where gaseous exchange does not occur
    D The space between the outside of the lung and the thoracic wall

101. The basic breathing cycle is controlled by respiratory centres in the brain. Where are these located?

A Hindbrain
B Midbrain
C Thalamus
D Cerebrum

102. Which statement is untrue?

A Overinflation of the lungs is prevented by the Hering-Breuer reflex
B The Hering-Breuer reflex is mediated via the vagus nerve
C Levels of oxygen are the most important factor in determining the rate of respiration
D The apneustic and pneumotaxic respiratory centres control expiration

103. The term that describes the total amount of air that is exhaled during forceful expiration after maximum inspiration is

A Tidal volume
B Residual volume
C Functional residual capacity
D Vital capacity

The digestive system

104. Which term means to pick up food?

A Prehension
B Deglutition
C Peristalsis
D Egestion

105. The philtrum is

A The point where the upper and lower lips meet
B The cleft in the upper lip
C The piece of tissue that is found under the tongue linking it to the floor of the mouth
D The gum

106. How many pairs of salivary glands does the dog have?

A 2
B 3
C 4
D 5

107. The correct dental formula for a kitten is

A I 3/3 C 1/1 PM 3/3
B I 3/3 C 1/1 PM 4/4 M 2/3
C I 3/3 C 1/1 PM 3/2
D I 3/3 C 1/1 PM 3/2 M 1/1

108. The region of the stomach closest to the oesophagus is the

A Pylorus
B Cardia
C Fundus
D Lesser curvature

109. The double fold of peritoneum that specifically links the stomach to the abdominal wall is called the

A Omentum
B Mesentery
C Ligament
D Serosa

110. Hydrochloric acid is secreted in the stomach to aid digestion and to protect the intestine from bacteria. Which cells in the stomach secrete this?

A Goblet cells
B Chief cells
C Parietal cells
D Beta cells

111. Into which part of the intestines does the gall bladder empty?

A Jejunum
B Ileum
C Duodenum
D Caecum

112. What is contained within the lacteals?

A Chyle
B Chyme
C Bile
D Proteins

113. Of the following, which is an enzyme used to break down proteins in the small intestine?

A Amylase
B Trypsin
C Pepsin
D Lipase

114. **The section of the intestine that absorbs water in the dog and cat is the**

    A Colon
    B Caecum
    C Ileum
    D Jejunum

115. **The liver is an important organ of the body carrying out several vital roles. Which of the following is not a function of the liver?**

    A Deamination of surplus amino acids
    B Synthesis of vitamins, including vitamins A and D
    C Fat metabolism
    D Destruction of old red blood cells

The urinary system

116. In which part of the kidney are the glomeruli found?

A Pelvis
B Medulla
C Cortex
D Capsule

117. The indentation on the side of the kidney where the renal blood vessels and ureter emerge is called the

A Calyx
B Hilus
C Apex
D Pyramid

118. In which order does fluid flow through the nephron as it is modified to form urine?

A Proximal convoluted tubule, distal convoluted tubule, loop of Henle, collecting duct
B Collecting duct, proximal convoluted tubule, loop of Henle, distal convoluted tubule
C Loop of Henle, proximal convoluted tubule, distal convoluted tubule, collecting duct
D Proximal convoluted tubule, loop of Henle, distal convoluted tubule, collecting duct

119. Sodium is only reabsorbed by the distal convoluted tubule of the kidney in the presence of which hormone?

A Aldosterone
B Angiotensin
C Renin
D Erythropoetin

120. Where is anti-diuretic hormone produced?

A Adrenal medulla
B Anterior pituitary
C Renal collecting ducts
D Posterior pituitary

121. **What is the unusual property of transitional epithelium compared with other epithelia of the body?**

    A It is permeable to certain substances
    B It is always stratified
    C It has the ability to close down around any tears in the tissue to prevent leakage
    D It is elastic and is able to stretch

122. **Under what conditions does the kidney secrete the hormone renin?**

    A High sodium levels
    B Low blood pressure
    C High levels of angiotensin
    D Low blood pH

123. **Urine flow through the ureter to the bladder is driven by**

    A Gravity
    B The ciliated mucous membrane lining the ureter
    C Peristaltic contractions of smooth muscle
    D Hydrostatic pressure

124. **There are two bladder sphincters involved in micturition. Which of the following statements is untrue?**

    A Parasympathetic neurons stimulate the reflex contraction of the bladder
    B Somatic motor neurons control the outer sphincter
    C Sympathetic neurons are involved in the process of micturition and stimulate bladder contraction
    D The nerves that are particularly important for bladder control are the sacral spinal nerves

The reproductive system

125. Spermatozoa are produced in which region of the male reproductive tract?

A   Epididymis
B   Deferent duct
C   Seminiferous tubules
D   Spermatic cord

126. The cells of Leydig (interstitial cells) produce which of the following?

A   Testosterone
B   Spermatozoa
C   Nutrients
D   Oestrogen

127. The spermatic cord runs from the testis into the abdomen. Which structure does not form part of this?

A   Cremaster muscle
B   Deferent duct
C   Spermatic nerve
D   Efferent tubule

128. The seminal fluid produced by the accessory glands in the male has a number of functions. However, which of the following is untrue about its role?

A   It increases the volume of the ejaculate
B   It increases survival time for the spermatozoa
C   It carries enzymes needed for fertilisation
D   It neutralises the acidity of the urine within the urethra

129. The statement about the penis in the male dog or cat that is untrue is

A   The tom's penis is directed caudally, and has tiny barbs covering the tip of the glans penis
B   The dog has an os penis, but the cat does not
C   The erectile tissue in the penis is called the corpus cavernosum penis
D   The urethra runs ventral to the os penis in the dog

130. **A female animal pregnant with her first litter can be described as**

    A Uniparous
    B Primigravid
    C Monoestrous
    D Multiparous

131. **The hormone needed to trigger ovulation is**

    A Progesterone
    B Oestrogen
    C Follicle stimulating hormone
    D Luteinising hormone

132. **The broad ligament covers part of the female reproductive tract. What is the name of the section that lies over the uterine tube or oviduct?**

    A Mesometrium
    B Mesosalpinx
    C Mesovarium
    D Mesoureter

133. **Which hormone *always* has an inhibitory effect on the release of follicle stimulating hormone from the pituitary?**

    A Progesterone
    B Oestrogen
    C Gonadotrophin releasing hormone
    D Luteinising hormone

134. **The infundibulum is found in which part of the female reproductive tract?**

    A At the distal end of the vestibule
    B At the proximal end of the uterine horn
    C At the proximal end of the uterine tube (oviduct)
    D At the junction of the uterine horns with the body of the uterus

135. Where is the external urethral orifice located?

A Adjacent to the cervix
B In the body of the uterus
C Close to the vulva
D In the floor of the vagina

136. During which stage of the oestrous cycle is the cervix open?

A Pro-oestrus
B Oestrus
C Metoestrus
D Anoestrus

137. The most accurate statement about the oestrous cycle of the queen is

A The queen is a spontaneous ovulator
B The queen is a seasonal breeder
C The queen is monoestrous
D Oestrus in the queen lasts 3 weeks

138. During which stage of the oestrous cycle may false pregnancy develop in the bitch?

A Pro-oestrus
B Oestrus
C Metoestrus
D Anoestrus

139. Mammary glands are which of the following types of glands?

A Modified sebaceous glands
B Modified apocrine glands
C Modified merocrine glands
D Modified endocrine glands

140. What is a zygote?

A   A fertilised ovum
B   A sperm or ovum
C   The developing young animal before its species is recognisable
D   The developing young animal after its species is recognisable

141. When does implantation of the blastocysts take place in the bitch?

A   7-10 days after ovulation
B   10-15 days after ovulation
C   14-20 days after ovulation
D   20-25 days after ovulation

142. The fluid-filled sac that lies closest to the developing embryo and cushions the foetus during delivery is the

A   Allantois
B   Amnion
C   Yolk sac
D   Chorion

143. Cats and dogs have which type of placenta?

A   Zonary placenta
B   Diffuse placenta
C   Discoid placenta
D   Cotyledonous placenta

The integument

144. **The cells of which layer of the skin have no nuclei and are fully keratinised?**

    A Stratum basale or germinativum
    B Stratum granulosum
    C Stratum lucidum
    D Stratum corneum

145. **Of the following types of glands, which are only found on the pads of the feet?**

    A Merocrine glands
    B Apocrine glands
    C Sebaceous glands
    D Meibomian glands

146. **Moulting of the hair coat is controlled by a number of different factors. Which of the following is not involved?**

    A Environmental temperature
    B Day length
    C Hormones
    D Grooming

147. **The type of hair attached to the arrector pili muscle, such that it can be raised if the animal is cold or frightened, is the**

    A Guard hair
    B Wool hair
    C Secondary hair
    D Vibrissa

148. **How many pads does the cat have on its forelimb?**

    A 4
    B 5
    C 6
    D 7

149. Cat claws are held in the retracted position by

A Smooth muscle
B Elastic ligaments
C Skeletal muscles
D Fibrous ligaments

The answers are on page 132

2 Observation and care of the patient

18 Questions

1. **Stress can hinder the recovery of hospitalised patients. Which of the following is not a suitable method for reducing stress in patients?**

   A   Place a male dog in close proximity to a bitch in season
   B   Provide individual care for each patient by one nurse
   C   Provide cats with somewhere to hide
   D   Provide adequate opportunity for urination and defaecation

2. **You are checking in-patients at the first morning check, and you observe the following cases. Which would give you cause for concern?**

   A   A dog with a capillary refill time of 1 second
   B   A rabbit passing a dark reddish urine
   C   A cat not interested in food
   D   A dog with a temperature of 103°F or 39.4°C

3. **The term that describes a depraved appetite in which a patient may crave unnatural foods is**

   A   Pica
   B   Anorexia
   C   Coprophagia
   D   Dysphagia

4. **What is the normal urine output for a dog?**

   A   0.5 ml/kg/hour
   B   1-2 ml/kg/hour
   C   5-10 ml/kg/hour
   D   10-20 ml/kg/hour

5. **Vaginal discharges in the bitch may occur for a number of reasons. Which of the following types is always abnormal?**

   A Bloody
   B Straw coloured
   C Dark green/brown
   D Cream

6. **In which situation might you see petechiae?**

   A In an animal suffering from anaemia
   B In an animal suffering from respiratory obstruction
   C In an animal with a bleeding disorder
   D In an animal suffering from jaundice

7. **Which is the correct formula for converting degrees Fahrenheit into degrees Centigrade?**

   A $(°F \div 5) \times 9 - 32$
   B $(°F - 32) \times 5 \div 9$
   C $(°F \times 9 \div 5) + 32$
   D $(°F + 32) \times 5 \div 9$

8. **If the rectal route cannot be used for measuring body temperature, what other location could be used?**

   A Sublingual
   B Frontal bone region (forehead)
   C External ear canal
   D Between the digits

9. **For how long should respirations be counted in order to determine respiratory rate?**

   A 15 seconds
   B 30 seconds
   C 1 minute
   D 5 minutes

10. **Which term means the same as poikilothermic?**

    A Endothermic
    B Ectothermic
    C Diathermic
    D Biothermic

11. **Decubitus ulcers can be prevented by which of the following methods?**

    A Massage limbs and skin regularly
    B Turn every 4 hours unless contraindicated
    C Use thick padding for animals that are unable to move easily
    D All of the above

12. **In the case of a burn, which type of dressing would be most appropriate to use?**

    A Dry dressing
    B Haemostatic dressing
    C Petroleum jelly impregnated gauze dressing
    D Saline soaked swabs

13. **For which situation would you apply a Velpeau sling?**

    A After a shoulder luxation
    B After a hip luxation
    C After a carpal luxation
    D After cruciate ligament disruption

14. **The absorption and effect of a medicine is slowest if given by which of the following routes?**

    A Orally
    B Intramuscular injection
    C Intraperitoneal injection
    D Subcutaneous injection

15. **Heat should be applied to improve wound healing in which of the following situations?**

    A Haemorrhage
    B Burns
    C Scalds
    D Abscesses

16. **How long does it take for an intramuscular injection to take effect?**

    A 30-45 minutes
    B 20-30 minutes
    C 0-2 minutes
    D Over 1 hour

17. **Intramuscular injections are often carried out into the quadriceps femoris muscle. Which other site is suitable?**

    A Gluteal muscles
    B Hamstrings muscles
    C Anterior tibial muscles
    D Lumbodorsal muscles

18. **For which products should you not wipe the top of the vial with an alcohol swab before drawing up the injection?**

    A Hormones
    B Antibiotics
    C Diuretics
    D Tranquillisers

The answers are on page 181

3 First aid

24 Questions

1. **The word triage refers to**

   A First aid treatment
   B Prioritising cases for treatment
   C Follow-up treatments once the first aid is completed
   D Bandaging wounds

2. **An emergency patient arrives at the surgery. Which of the following is the most important thing to assess?**

   A Bleeding
   B Shock
   C Airway
   D Colour of mucous membranes

3. **A client calls for advice about transporting an injured dog to the surgery. Which is the least appropriate advice to give?**

   A If a dog is able to walk, then it should be allowed to do so, however slowly
   B Animals with suspected abdominal injuries should be carried by stretcher
   C The best type of stretcher for an animal other than a commercial animal stretcher is a blanket
   D A muzzle should be used when transferring a conscious animal onto a stretcher

4. **The term strabismus means which of the following?**

   A Rapid flickering of the eyes
   B One pupil is smaller than the other
   C A squint
   D Abnormal papillary reflexes

5. **The clinical signs of shock include all of the following except**

   A Increased respiration rate
   B Weak rapid pulse
   C Cold extremities
   D Decreased capillary refill time

6. **In which of the following cases might it be appropriate to give a hypertonic solution intravenously to a patient?**

   A A dog with severe vomiting and diarrhoea
   B A cat with a head injury leading to compression of the brain
   C A cat with extensive blood loss
   D A dog in shock

7. **If you are attempting cardio-pulmonary resuscitation on your own, which resuscitation protocol is recommended?**

   A 1 breath every 5 cardiac compressions
   B 2 breaths every 10 cardiac compressions
   C 1 breath every 10 cardiac compressions
   D 2 breaths every 15 cardiac compressions

8. **With which of the following conditions might a cat show hindlimb paralysis with cold toes?**

   A Arterial thromboembolism
   B Fractured femur
   C Shock
   D Hypothermia

9. **Pregnancy and parturition can be a worrying time for owners of a bitch or queen. If a client called about one of the following animals, which would you advise should be seen by a vet as soon as possible?**

   A A bitch that has started showing signs of restlessness and nest making, but has not produced a pup after 4 hours of this behaviour
   B A pregnant bitch that shows a green-brown discharge, but has not shown any signs of starting to whelp
   C A cat that has delivered three kittens, but has stopped for an over an hour, though more kittens are expected. No signs of straining are being shown
   D A bitch due to whelp that has shown a drop in temperature 12 hours ago, but is only just starting to show signs of intermittent straining

10. **Which method is the least suitable to use when resuscitating neonates?**

   A Dislodge fluid from the airways by swinging the young while supporting the head and neck
   B Dry the neonate by vigorously rubbing it with a towel
   C Use doxapram drops under the tongue to stimulate respiration under the veterinary surgeon's direction
   D Intermittent positive pressure ventilation using an anaesthetic circuit and oxygen

11. **Hypocalcaemia due to pregnancy or lactation is also referred to as**

   A Eclampsia
   B Paraphimosis
   C Pyometra
   D Pseudocyesis

12. **An owner has called to say that her dog has just started to fit. Which advice would be inappropriate to give her?**

   A Darken the room
   B Move objects away from the animal
   C Ensure that its tongue is pulled forward
   D Turn off televisions or radios

13. **The condition that might result in an animal showing pollakiuria is**

    A Cystitis
    B Parvovirus infection
    C Peritonitis
    D Severe dehydration

14. **If an animal was collapsed, with sweet-smelling breath, which disease condition would you suspect?**

    A Diabetes mellitus
    B Addison's disease
    C Hypoglycaemia
    D Hypocalcaemia

15. **Which of the following conditions could be life threatening?**

    A Fractured femur
    B Prolapsed eye
    C Bee sting
    D Aural haematoma

16. **The first action you should take if an animal was thought to have ingested paraquat is to**

    A Give a demulcent
    B Induce emesis
    C Keep it warm
    D Wash the coat

17. **A dog has been presented at the surgery with acute paraphimosis. Which of the following first aid treatments would be suitable?**

    A Hot compress application
    B Ice pack application
    C Irrigation with cold water
    D Antiseptic irrigation

18. **The poison that can cause central blindness is**

    A Lead
    B Organophosphates
    C Metaldehyde
    D Blue-green algae

19. **The body naturally deals with haemorrhage in four ways. These include all of the following except**

    A Production of inflammatory mediators such as histamine
    B Retraction of the damaged ends of blood vessels
    C Back pressure
    D Blood clotting

20. **What would you do initially to control haemorrhage from a large wound to the proximal thigh in which there could be a foreign body?**

    A Apply pressure to the brachial pressure point
    B Apply direct pressure
    C Apply a tourniquet
    D Apply indirect pressure

21. **Burns caused by which of the following are usually the slowest to show the severity of the damage?**

    A Dry heat
    B Hot fats or oils
    C Extreme cold
    D Moist heat

22. **Emesis is often indicated as a first aid measure for poisoning. Which of the following methods should not be used?**

    A Concentrated salt solution orally
    B Washing soda crystals orally
    C Apomorphine injection, under veterinary direction
    D Concentrated mustard solution orally

23. **A fracture in which there are several fracture fragments is described as**

    A Multiple
    B Complicated
    C Compound
    D Comminuted

24. **The first aid management for a luxation is to**

    A Reduce the luxation as soon as possible
    B Apply heat to the area
    C Restrict movement of the affected joint
    D All of the above

The answers are on page 186

4 Animal handling and basic animal management

22 Questions

1. **Which statement is true concerning the restraint of animals?**

   A Cats should always be blindfolded to reduce aggression
   B Rabbits should be handled by the ears and scruff
   C A rolled up towel can be used to restrain the head of a brachycephalic dog
   D A rat should be picked up by the base of the tail

2. **Of the following methods, which should only be used as a last resort when restraining a dog?**

   A Dog catcher
   B Basket muzzle
   C Tape muzzle
   D Hold the scruff either side of the neck

3. **A dog you are about to handle wags its tail as you approach it. Which best describes your interpretation of its behaviour?**

   A It is happy and will be easy to handle
   B All animals showing this are going to be very difficult to handle due to aggression
   C You are still wary since nervous or aggressive dogs may also show this
   D This dog is terrified, and is going to need a lot of reassurance

4. **If you are approaching a nervous dog, which of the following should not be carried out?**

    A Let the dog come to you first, rather than directly approaching the dog
    B Make prolonged eye contact
    C Keep hands low, and fingers curled inwards whilst approaching
    D Move slowly and deliberately

5. **If a dog growls at you, which is the most appropriate course of action?**

    A Comfort and reassure the dog
    B Punish the dog by shouting at it
    C Back off immediately
    D Muzzle the dog

6. **Some dogs are fine on arrival at the surgery but become aggressive when someone tries to remove them from the safety of the kennel. If you have an animal known to show this behaviour, which of the following approaches would not be suitable to use?**

    A The dog should be tied up outside a kennel
    B A lead should be left on the dog with the end left outside the kennel
    C A choke chain should be used, with a lead attached to this and the kennel door
    D The kennel should be opened and the dog allowed to come forward and a slip lead then placed on the dog

7. **Minimum and maximum temperatures recommended for animals in 'Model Licence Conditions and Guidance for Dog Boarding Establishments' are**

    A 10°C - 26°C
    B 4°C - 20°C
    C 14°C - 22°C
    D 6°C - 30°C

8. **Since cats like to climb, what is the minimum recommended height for a unit within a boarding cattery?**

   A 0.6 m (2 ft)
   B 1.2 m (4 ft)
   C 1.8 m (6 ft)
   D 2.1 m (8 ft)

9. **Passive ventilation would be provided by**

   A Ventilation bricks
   B Extractor fans
   C Air-conditioning systems
   D Wood-wool insulation

10. **A wound could be cleansed with which type of product?**

    A Biguanide
    B Peroxide
    C Hypochlorite
    D Aldehyde

11. **Which of the following is a phenolic disinfectant?**

    A Halogenated tertiary amine
    B Glutaraldehyde
    C Chloroxylenol
    D Povidone-iodine

12. **A quaternary ammonium compound such as cetrimide is a/n**

    A Anionic surfactant
    B Cationic surfactant
    C Amphoteric surfactant
    D Non-ionic surfactant

13. **In-patient care is an important part of nursing. Which statement is incorrect about the need to groom in-patients?**

    A Grooming should be considered a part of all in-patients' care
    B Grooming allows nursing staff the opportunity to check the animal's body more closely
    C Grooming is unnecessary for short-haired animals
    D Grooming may improve the animal's feeling of well-being and promote recovery

14. **Dental care is carried out by many owners. However, which statement is actually true?**

    A Animal or human toothpaste can be used without problem
    B Animal toothbrushes are the same as human ones
    C Finger stall toothbrushes may be useful to introduce animals to the sensation of bristles
    D A mouthwash can be used instead of brushing the teeth

15. **When might veterinary staff use a styptic?**

    A To remove mats from a tangled coat
    B To examine the ear of an animal
    C To control mild haemorrhage
    D To remove a tick from the animal's skin

16. **The quarantine period for animals entering the UK that are not covered by the Pet Travel Scheme (PETS) is**

    A 2 months
    B 6 months
    C 9 months
    D 1 year

17. **If an owner wishes their animal to travel abroad under PETS, all of the following are true except**

   A   The animal must be vaccinated against rabies, and the animal blood tested to be sure the vaccine provides sufficient protection

   B   Treatment against tapeworm and ticks should be carried out 24-48 hours before return to the UK

   C   The animal must be tattooed with permanent identification

   D   Only certain entry points to the UK can accept animals travelling under the scheme

18. **Cats and dogs are not the only species subject to quarantine requirements. Other species that are not exempt include**

   A   Primates

   B   Horses

   C   Guinea pigs

   D   Sheep

19. **The Dangerous Dogs Act 1991 (amended 1997) prohibits the ownership of certain breeds of dogs in the UK. This includes all of the following except**

   A   Japanese Tosa

   B   Pit Bull Terrier

   C   Dogo Argentino

   D   Dogue de Bordeaux

20. **What is the name of the organisation that recognises and classifies pedigree cat breeds in the UK?**

   A   The Cattery Club

   B   The Governing Council of Cat Fancy

   C   Feline Advisory Bureau

   D   Show Cat Council

21. **The piece of grooming equipment suitable to use on a short-coated breed of dog such as a Weimaraner is a**

   A   Slicker brush

   B   Hound glove

   C   Rake

   D   Pin brush

22. **The Kennel Club recognises 7 groups of dogs, and these are divided into Sporting and Non-Sporting. Which group would be described as Non-Sporting?**

    A Working group
    B Hound group
    C Gundog group
    D Terrier group

The answers are on page 193

5 Practice organisation, management, law and ethics

15 Questions

1. **A written statement of a business's purpose is described as its**

    A Mission statement
    B Business plan
    C Financial plan
    D SWOT analysis

2. **The statement relating to the reception area and communication skills that is untrue is**

    A Reception staff are often the first point of contact for a client, and it is therefore important that a favourable impression is created
    B Body language can be as important as verbal communication when dealing with clients
    C More clients are lost as a result of their animal dying at the surgery than due to poor communication skills of veterinary staff
    D The reason for a client wishing to make an appointment should be checked, since this will influence the length of consultation required

3. **Data stored by practices about clients and employees is subject to controls. Which of the statements about this is correct?**

   A Clients have no right to access records of their animals, since the records are the property of the practice

   B All practices have to register with the Data Protection Registrar under the Data Protection Act 1984

   C All case records must be kept for 6 years and 364 days

   D Practices must keep employee PAYE details for at least 3 years

4. **The monitor of a computer is described by which acronym?**

   A CPU

   B VDU

   C CD-ROM

   D RAM

5. **The true statement about active clients and bonded clients is that**

   A An active client is defined as one whose pet's vaccinations have been kept up to date

   B A bonded client is one who has visited the practice within the last few years

   C An active client is one who has visited the practice within a given period of time

   D Active and bonded clients are two terms for the same thing

6. **Which Schedule of the Veterinary Surgeons Act 1966 allows a qualified listed veterinary nurse to undertake minor acts of surgery?**

   A Schedule 1

   B Schedule 2

   C Schedule 3

   D Schedule 4

7. **Which Act is an 'enabling Act'?**

   A Veterinary Surgeons Act 1966
   B Health and Safety At Work Act 1974
   C Data Protection Act 1984
   D Dangerous Dogs Act 1991

8. **A minor civil law case is usually heard in the**

   A County Court
   B Magistrates Court
   C Crown Court
   D High Court

9. **Under current systems of work, who is accountable for the actions of a qualified, listed veterinary nurse who is a member of the British Veterinary Nursing Association?**

   A The BVNA
   B The veterinary surgeon
   C The veterinary nurse
   D The RCVS

10. **Under the Health and Safety at Work Act 1974, which persons are protected?**

    A The employer
    B The employees
    C Visitors to the workplace
    D All the above

11. **Of the following pieces of legislation, which does not deal with the safe disposal of waste?**

    A Control of Pollution Act 1974
    B Controlled Waste Regulations 1992
    C Environmental Protection Act 1990
    D Control of Substances Hazardous to Health Regulations 1999

12. **The type of waste that must be placed into rigid yellow plastic tubs, and then collected and incinerated by an authorised company, is**

    A Clinical waste
    B Special waste
    C Cadavers
    D Non-clinical commercial waste

13. **Which of the following accidents or illnesses that might occur in a veterinary surgery would not normally need to be reported to the Health and Safety Executive under the provisions of RIDDOR 1995?**

    A A student nurse falling off a stool and fracturing her arm
    B A client being bitten by her cat
    C A veterinary surgeon developing leptospirosis after dealing with a case
    D An oxygen cylinder exploding

14. **In risk assessments, what does MEL stand for?**

    A Minimum environmental levels
    B Maximum engineering load
    C Minimum essential layers
    D Maximum exposure limits

15. **If a chemical was labelled with this symbol, what would this indicate?**

    A Toxic
    B Highly flammable
    C Corrosive
    D Harmful

The answers are on page 199

6 Nutrition

21 Questions

1. **Taurine deficiency in cats could lead to which of the following problems?**

   A Weight loss
   B Skeletal abnormalities
   C Dilated cardiomyopathy
   D Scurfy skin

2. **The true statement about dietary fats is that**

   A Fats have a lower calorific content per gram than protein
   B There are four essential fatty acids
   C Fats are important in the diet as carriers of the fat-soluble vitamins
   D Most dietary fats are made of glycerol combined with a fatty acid molecule

3. **The disease condition unrelated to lack of calcium is**

   A Hyperthyroidism
   B Rickets
   C Hyperparathyroidism
   D Eclampsia

4. **Lack of potassium in the bloodstream is described as**

   A Hyponatraemia
   B Hypocupraemia
   C Hypokalaemia
   D Hypocalcaemia

5. **The trace element which has an anti-oxidant function in the body, and works in conjunction with vitamin E is**

   A Iron
   B Iodine
   C Manganese
   D Selenium

6. **When referring to proteins, biological value is a measure of**

   A Their calorific value
   B Both the digestibility and quality of the protein
   C Its availability in foods
   D The ease with which the protein can be used for other purposes within the body

7. **Vitamin A is also known as**

   A Calciferol
   B Thiamin
   C Ascorbic acid
   D Retinol

8. **Of the following vitamins, which is fat soluble?**

   A Vitamin C
   B Vitamin B_6
   C Vitamin K
   D Niacin

9. **The name given to water generated through chemical reactions within the body is**

   A Metabolic water
   B Chemical water
   C Total body water
   D Interstitial water

10. **What is the problem with feeding raw egg?**

   A It contains thiaminases, which break down vitamin B_1
   B It contains phytates, which prevent the absorption of zinc
   C It contains very high levels of vitamin A, which can lead to hypervitaminosis A
   D It contains avidin, which binds biotin, and reduces its availability

11. **The nutritional requirements of cats are not quite the same as those of dogs. Which statement is true about the needs of each species?**

    A Cats have only a limited ability to break down carbohydrates, which makes them intolerant of high carbohydrate diets

    B Dogs are obligate carnivores

    C Cats are able to convert β-carotene to vitamin A (retinol)

    D Dog food can be fed to cats instead of cat food, providing it is of good quality

12. **When feeding a bitch during pregnancy, which of the following protocols would be suitable?**

    A Feed additional amounts of a concentrated diet from the day of mating so that she has sufficient nutrients to meet the pups' needs

    B Supplements of calcium and vitamin D should be given throughout the pregnancy

    C Food should only be increased during the later stages of pregnancy (from 5th/6th week)

    D Lactating bitches usually require less food than a bitch in the late stages of pregnancy

13. **Puppies fed imbalanced diets are particularly at risk from developmental skeletal abnormalities. All the nutrients below are implicated in causing problems except**

    A Vitamin C

    B Calcium

    C Vitamin A

    D Vitamin D

14. **What weight should a kitten have reached by the time it is weaned?**

    A 300 g - 500 g

    B 600 g - 1000 g

    C 1.2 kg - 1.5 kg

    D Over 1.5 kg

15. **The untrue statement about the dietary needs of older cats and dogs is**

    A Older cats should have a reduced calorie intake compared with when they were younger
    B Protein sources for older animals should have a high biological value
    C Phosphorus levels may need to be restricted in animals with renal disease
    D Sodium restriction is beneficial in animals with cardiac problems

16. **The most common presenting sign in animals with dietary sensitivity is**

    A Diarrhoea
    B Pruritus and self-trauma
    C Vomiting
    D Gastric dilation

17. **One way to check if an animal has a dietary sensitivity is to use a restriction diet. How long should this be tried for?**

    A At least 2 weeks
    B At least 3 weeks
    C At least a month
    D At least 3 months

18. **Rapid weight loss in obese cats can lead to which of the following conditions?**

    A Diabetes mellitus
    B Feline lower urinary tract disease
    C Osteoarthritis
    D Hepatic lipidosis

19. **Coconut oil is a good source of dietary medium chain triglycerides. In which type of problem would this form of fat be useful?**

    A Malabsorption
    B Colitis
    C Diabetes mellitus
    D Pancreatitis

20. **Calcium oxalate crystal formation may lead to urolithiasis. Which statement is true about the management of this condition?**

    A The uroliths can be dissolved by feeding a diet which has an acidifying effect on the urine
    B It is not possible to actually dissolve calcium oxalate uroliths by dietary modification
    C This condition occurs mostly in Dalmatians
    D Restriction of protein in the diet and the administration of allopurinol can prevent recurrence of this condition

21. **The mineral lost in urine during prolonged use of frusemide diuretics is**

    A Calcium
    B Sodium
    C Chloride
    D Potassium

The answers are on page 204

7 Genetics and animal breeding

12 Questions

1. **The name given to the chromosomes in the nucleus that are not the X and Y chromosomes is**

   A Sex chromosomes
   B Autosomes
   C Alleles
   D Homosomes

2. **Sex-limited and sex-linked are terms used to describe two different genetic principles. Which statement is true about these?**

   A Sex-linked genes are only found on the Y chromosome
   B Sex-limited genes are only expressed in one sex
   C Sex-limited genes are found on the X and Y chromosomes
   D Sex-linked genes confer the sexual characteristics of animals

3. **The term that describes an animal which has two different alleles for the same gene is**

   A Homozygous
   B Homologous
   C Hemizygous
   D Heterozygous

4. **If two heterozygous animals are mated, what proportion of their offspring should show the recessive characteristic?**

   A All of the young
   B Half of the young
   C A quarter of the young
   D None of the young

5. **The external appearance of an animal is termed its**

   A Genotype
   B Phenotype
   C Epistasis
   D Epistaxis

6. **Which is the correct sequence of events during mitosis?**

   A Prophase, metaphase, anaphase, telophase
   B Anaphase, prophase, metaphase, telophase
   C Prophase, anaphase, telophase, metaphase
   D Metaphase, prophase, telophase, anaphase

7. **Of the following, which can also be referred to as a gamete?**

   A A fertilised egg
   B A stem cell
   C An ovum
   D An altered gene

8. **What is meant by the F1 generation?**

   A This refers to the animals that are about to be mated
   B This refers to the parents of animals about to be mated
   C This refers to the siblings of animals about to be mated
   D This refers to the offspring of animals about to be mated

9. **Of the following pairs of genes, which are most likely to show linkage?**

   A Two genes on the same chromosome
   B A gene on the X chromosome and a gene on an autosome
   C A gene on two different autosomes
   D A gene on the X chromosome and a gene on the Y chromosome

10. **Two animals are mated that are less closely related than if selected at random. What is the term given to this form of breeding?**

    A Inbreeding
    B Outbreeding
    C Line breeding
    D Random breeding

11. **An abnormality or defect present at birth can be described as a/n**

    A Mutation
    B Phenocopy
    C Inherited defect
    D Congenital defect

12. **In which species of dog might you see copper toxicosis resulting from an inherited defect?**

    A Irish Setters
    B German Shepherd Dogs
    C Bedlington Terriers
    D West Highland White Terriers

The answers are on page 210

8 Exotic pets and wildlife

21 Questions

1. **Rabbits use bacteria to break down cellulose in their diet. In which part of the gastrointestinal tract does most of this process take place?**

   A Stomach
   B Small intestine
   C Large intestine
   D Caecum

2. **Which statement is true about gerbils?**

   A They have no pads on the feet
   B They may have a dewlap
   C They have a large skin gland on the mid-ventral abdomen
   D They have glandular areas on their flanks

3. **Canaries are members of which order of birds?**

   A Psittaciformes
   B Anseriformes
   C Galliformes
   D Passeriformes

4. **The number of digits a bird has in its wings is**

   A 1
   B 2
   C 3
   D 4

5. **The true statement about the crop in the bird's digestive tract is that**

    A It is the name for the glandular stomach
    B It is the organ in which food is stored prior to digestion
    C It is where seeds and coarse food are ground up
    D It is where most bacterial breakdown of plant material occurs

6. **Gaseous exchange take place in which tissues in birds?**

    A In the air sacs
    B In bones
    C In the abdomen
    D In the lungs

7. **When might an ectothermic animal aestivate?**

    A When temperatures are too low
    B When food is scarce
    C When temperatures are too high
    D When humidity is too high

8. **The species with only one functional lung is the**

    A Snake
    B Lizard
    C Tortoise
    D Toad

9. **The correct definition for the term ovo-viviparous is**

    A The females retain their eggs within their bodies until the young are ready to hatch
    B Eggs are laid which require incubation before the young are ready to hatch
    C Young animals are born after being nurtured by the mother via a placenta
    D Eggs are laid which are stored within the male until ready to hatch

10. **How much vitamin C does an adult guinea pig require per day?**

    A 10 mg
    B 20 mg
    C 30 mg
    D 50 mg

11. **Of the following species, which are induced ovulators?**

    A Rabbits
    B Guinea pigs
    C Chinchillas
    D Hamsters

12. **How long can a parrot live for?**

    A 10-15 years
    B 20-30 years
    C 30-40 years
    D 40-50 years

13. **Some birds of prey are protected from being held in captivity by the Wildlife and Countryside Act 1981. However, if the bird is under the care of a veterinary surgeon, it is exempt (providing that proper records are kept) for a period of**

    A 2 weeks
    B 4 weeks
    C 6 weeks
    D 8 weeks

14. **Which statement is incorrect about the care of tortoises?**

    A Tortoises should not be fed for 3-4 weeks prior to hibernation
    B Hermann's tortoise can be identified by the presence of a spur on the end of its tail
    C Healthy tortoises can lose up to 3% of their bodyweight per month during hibernation
    D Overfeeding young tortoises can lead to shell deformities

15. **The term that means shedding of the skin, as snakes do, is**

    A Ecdysis
    B Autotomy
    C Setae
    D Myiasis

16. **The disinfectant suitable to use on plants prior to adding them to an aquarium is**

    A Chlorhexidine solution
    B Povidone-iodine solution
    C Salt solution
    D Potassium permanganate solution

17. **The animals that may show 'barbering' are**

    A Rabbits
    B Guinea pigs
    C Rats
    D Hamsters

18. **Which disease seen in birds can also cause problems in humans?**

    A Psittacine beak and feather disease (PBFD)
    B Trichomoniasis
    C Newcastle disease
    D Psittacosis

19. **A blood sample for a tortoise should be collected from the**

    A Jugular vein
    B Cephalic vein
    C Ventral tail vein
    D Marginal ear vein

20. **For which species is Jackson's ratio a useful indicator of health?**

    A Tortoises
    B Birds
    C Fish
    D Snakes

21. Which of the following species require fasting prior to anaesthesia?

A Gerbils
B Tortoises
C Snakes
D Both snakes and tortoises

The answers are on page 214

9 Medicines: pharmacology, therapeutics and dispensing

17 Questions

1. **The therapeutic index of a drug is**

   A The ratio between the dose which causes toxic effects and the dose that provides the desired effect
   B The type of action the drug has in the body
   C The way in which the drug is absorbed, metabolised and excreted by the body
   D The dose of a drug that experimentally causes death in 50% of the animals tested

2. **Of the following descriptions, which best describes the action of bacteriostatic drugs?**

   A They kill bacteria
   B They kill all micro-organisms
   C They prevent multiplication of all micro-organisms
   D They prevent the multiplication of bacteria

3. **Which of the following drugs is used as an antiviral product?**

   A Nystatin
   B Acyclovir
   C Fenbendazole
   D Amoxycillin

4. **The drug used in cardiac disease that acts to increase the force of cardiac contraction is**

   A Lignocaine (Xylocaine)
   B Enalapril (Enacard)
   C Pimobendan (Vetmedin)
   D Propranolol (Inderal)

5. **The treatment or management of epilepsy can involve the use of**

   A Antimuscarinics
   B Muscle relaxants
   C Barbiturates
   D Local anaesthetics

6. **The non-steroidal anti-inflammatory drug licensed for use as part of a premedication in small animals is**

   A Phenylbutazone (PBZ)
   B Aspirin
   C Flunixin meglumine (Finadyne)
   D Carprofen (Zenecarp)

7. **Which products are used on skin to leave a protective covering of protein?**

   A Keratolytics
   B Astringents
   C Mucolytics
   D Mydriatics

8. **Of the following statements about drugs that act on the immune system, which is untrue?**

   A Vaccines contain altered or killed organisms
   B Toxoids contain preformed antibodies to toxins
   C Antisera contain preformed antibodies to organisms
   D Antitoxins and toxoids are not identical

9. **What is the concentration of a 1.25% solution in mg/ml?**

   A 1.25 mg/ml
   B 12.5 mg/ml
   C 125 mg/ml
   D 25 mg/ml

10. **Under the medicine cascade, which of the following products should be used as a last resort?**

    A A product which has no product license for animals or humans
    B A product that is licensed for use in the species to be treated but for a different condition
    C A product that is licensed for use in another species for the same condition
    D A product that is licensed for human use

11. **Which class of drugs dispensed in a veterinary surgery can be sold to someone without the vet having seen their animal?**

    A Pharmacy products
    B Pharmacy and Merchants List products
    C Prescription Only Medicines
    D General Sales List products

12. **Volumes of liquids for external use should be dispensed in**

    A A wide-mouthed jar
    B A glass or plastic container with a child-proof lid
    C A coloured fluted bottle
    D A coloured smooth bottle

13. **Legally, which of the following information is not essential on a label of a dispensed product?**

    A For Animal Treatment Only
    B Date
    C Quantity and strength of drug
    D Veterinary practice address

14. **The legislation that gives details about the use, storage and supply of Controlled Drugs is**

    A The Medicines Act 1968
    B Control of Substances Hazardous to Health Regulations 1999
    C The Health and Safety at Work Act 1974
    D The Misuse of Drugs Act 1971

15. **All the Controlled Drugs are classed into schedules according to the risk of addiction and abuse by humans. In which Schedule is diazepam?**

    A Schedule 1
    B Schedule 2
    C Schedule 3
    D Schedule 4

16. **How long should a Controlled Drug register be kept after the last entry?**

    A 1 year
    B 2 years
    C 5 years
    D 7 years

17. **The abbreviation used on a prescription that means every 8 hours is**

    A om
    B prn
    C q8h
    D tbs

The answers are on page 219

10 Laboratory diagnostic aids

24 Questions

1. **Which type of pipette should be used to transfer small volumes of fluid, for example to separate plasma from a blood sample after centrifugation?**

   A One mark volumetric pipette
   B Automatic pipette
   C Pasteur pipette
   D Graduated pipette

2. **The part of the microscope that holds the objective lenses is the**

   A Nosepiece
   B Mechanical stage
   C Condenser
   D Body

3. **The objective lens which can be referred to as the high dry lens is**

   A x4
   B x10
   C x20
   D x40

4. **What temperature is usually used for the incubation and culture of bacteria?**

   A 32°C
   B 34°C
   C 37°C
   D 40°C

5. **The anticoagulant that is best for blood samples that are to be used for haematological studies is**

   A Heparin
   B Ethylene diamine tetra-acetic acid (EDTA)
   C Sodium citrate
   D Fluoride oxalate

6. **If a urine sample is to be cultured for bacteria, which method of urine collection should be used?**

   A Mid-stream sample
   B Catheterisation
   C Cystocentesis
   D Manual expression

7. **When collecting a faeces sample which statement is incorrect?**

   A Samples should be collected directly from the rectum
   B The pot should be filled to a maximum of a quarter full
   C Faeces should be examined as soon as possible
   D If needed, urine collection should be carried out before faecal collection

8. **For which clinical condition would you use hair plucks for diagnosis?**

   A Yeasts
   B Mites
   C Bacteria
   D Ringworm

9. **The largest pathological fluid sample that can be sent in the post is**

   A 10 ml
   B 20 ml
   C 50 ml
   D 100 ml

10. **Blood smears can be stained using supra-vital stains. Which of the following is an example of this type of stain?**

    A Brilliant cresyl blue
    B Wright's stain
    C Leishman's stain
    D Giemsa stain

11. **What is the normal white blood cell count in a dog?**

    A 5.5-8.5 x 10^9/l
    B 6-18 x 10^9/l
    C 5.5-8.5 x 10^{12}/l
    D 6-18 x 10^{12}/l

12. **In which cells might you find Howell-Jolly bodies?**

    A Granulocytes
    B Monocytes
    C Reticulocytes
    D Lymphocytes

13. **The white cells usually seen in increased numbers in animals with viral conditions are**

    A Lymphocytes
    B Monocytes
    C Eosinophils
    D Neutrophils

14. **Biochemical tests are often run to screen animals for underlying disease. Which statement is true about some of the common tests?**

    A Blood urea nitrogen (BUN) and urea levels in blood are the same thing, and have the same value
    B Glucose levels are constant throughout the day
    C Alanine aminotransferase (ALT) is more liver specific in small animals than aspartate aminotransferase (AST)
    D Creatinine levels depend on both renal and hepatic function

15. **10% potassium hydroxide is often used in examination of skin scrapings. Why is it helpful?**

    A Potassium hydroxide fixes the scrapings, so that the sample can be kept and examined again at a later date
    B Potassium hydroxide stains the hair shafts, allowing easier visualisation of ringworm organisms
    C Potassium hydroxide shows up mites more clearly by highlighting them
    D Potassium hydroxide clears the slide of cellular debris, and makes it easier to examine hair shafts for evidence of ringworm or ectoparasites

16. **The stain used to show up undigested fat in a faecal smear is**

    A Sudan III
    B Lugol's iodine
    C Eosin
    D New methylene blue

17. **At what speed should urine samples be centrifuged for 5 minutes in order to separate sediment from supernatant?**

    A 500 rpm
    B 1,500 rpm
    C 3,000 rpm
    D 10,000 rpm

18. **How long does an animal need to be on a meat-free diet before its faeces can be tested for occult blood?**

    A 3 days
    B 5 days
    C 1 week
    D Over 1 week

19. A refractometer is used to take a urine specific gravity reading. The initial reading is off the scale, so the sample is diluted with the same volume of distilled water. The refractometer reading is now 1.032. What was the original reading?

    A 2.064
    B 1.016
    C 1.064
    D 1.096

20. Of the following, which may give false negatives for glucose if present in urine samples being tested by urine dipsticks?

    A Bleach
    B Ascorbic acid
    C Blood
    D Bilirubin

21. The crystal seen in urine that characteristically has a flat hexagonal appearance is

    A Cystine
    B Calcium oxalate
    C Ammonium urate
    D Struvite (ammonium triple phosphate)

22. Which stain is useful for demonstrating the presence of bacteria, without giving information about their Gram status?

    A Leishman's stain
    B Lugol's iodine
    C Eosin
    D Methylene blue

23. Of the following components of Gram's stain, which is described as the counterstain?

    A Crystal violet
    B Lugol's iodine
    C Acetone
    D Carbol fuschin

24. Which method for preserving urine would be best to use if the sample was to be tested for bacteriological growth?

A Acetic acid
B Hydrochloric acid
C Thymol crystal
D Boric acid

The answers are on page 225

11 Elementary microbiology and immunology

12 Questions

1. **The true statement about micro-organisms is that**

   A Parasitic micro-organisms are always pathogenic
   B Commensal organisms cause no harm or benefit to the host
   C All bacteria produce toxins
   D All infectious diseases are contagious

2. **The types of organism responsible for the production of endotoxins are**

   A Gram-negative bacteria
   B Gram-positive bacteria
   C Viruses
   D Fungi

3. **A disease normally present within an area can be described as**

   A Pandemic
   B Epidemic
   C Epizootic
   D Endemic

4. **Of the following, which is used to stimulate the development of an animal's immunity against a toxin?**

   A Toxoid
   B Antiserum
   C Vaccine
   D Antitoxin

5. **Bacteria with a curved rod shape can be classed as**

   A Bacilli
   B Vibrios
   C Cocci
   D Spirochaetes

6. **The term that best describes a bacterium that grows best in the presence of oxygen but will grow (more slowly) in its absence is**

   A Facultative aerobe
   B Obligate anaerobe
   C Microaerophile
   D Facultative anaerobe

7. **Of the following, which genus of bacteria produce spores?**

   A Escherichia
   B Streptococcus
   C Clostridium
   D Salmonella

8. **What is conjugation?**

   A A form of sexual reproduction seen in some bacteria
   B Fusion of two bacteria to produce one super bacterium
   C A means by which genetic information may be transferred from one bacterium to another
   D Bacterial replication

9. **Which of the following media encourages the growth of Salmonella whilst inhibiting other bacteria?**

   A Deoxycholate citrate agar
   B MacConkey agar
   C Blood agar
   D Chocolate agar

10. **Which of the following is true about viruses?**

   A Viruses contain both RNA and DNA
   B Viruses are either icosahedral or helical in shape
   C Viruses always contain nucleic acid and a protein coat
   D Viruses with envelopes are always helical

11. **The type of organism thought to be the cause of Feline Spongiform Encephalopathy is a**

    A Prion
    B Virus
    C Fungus
    D Bacterium

12. **Host immunity can be divided into non-specific immunity and specific immunity. Which of the following is an example of non-specific immunity?**

    A Antibody production
    B Lymphokine production
    C Cell-mediated immunity
    D Interferon

The answers are on page 232

12 Elementary mycology and parasitology

20 Questions

1. **Of the following fungi, which is responsible for cases of ringworm in small animals?**

   A Malassezia pachydermatis
   B Candida albicans
   C Aspergillus fumigatus
   D Trichophyton mentagrophytes

2. **The medium suitable for culturing fungi is**

   A MacConkey agar
   B Sabouraud's medium
   C Blood agar
   D Chocolate agar

3. **For which parasite is the larval form the only parasitic stage?**

   A Felicola subrostratus
   B Trombicula autumnalis
   C Ctenocephalides felis
   D Sarcoptes scabiei

4. **The sucking louse of the dog is**

   A Felicola subrostratus
   B Linognathus setosus
   C Trichodectes setosus
   D Damalinia bovis

5. **Pediculosis is a term used to describe a type of parasitic infestation. Which of the following parasites would cause this?**

   A Fleas
   B Ticks
   C Blow fly maggots
   D Lice

6. **Flea infestations can cause a number of problems. Which of the following is not true about possible consequences of flea infestations?**

   A Fleas may carry Haemobartonella felis and transfer the disease feline infectious anaemia
   B Fleas may carry Taenia hydatigena, and transfer the tapeworm
   C Fleas may cause anaemia
   D Fleas can cause allergic dermatitis in the infested animal

7. **Which of the following is an insect?**

   A Ctenocephalides canis
   B Sarcoptes scabiei
   C Demodex canis
   D Trichophyton mentagrophytes

8. **The parasite that is not host specific is**

   A Demodex canis
   B Trichodectes canis
   C Notoedres cati
   D Ctenocephalides felis

9. **The mite responsible for scaly leg in cage birds is**

   A Notoedres
   B Cnemidocoptes
   C Demodex
   D Trixacarus

10. 'Walking dandruff' is the nickname given to which surface-living mite?

   A Trombicula
   B Otodectes
   C Cheyletiella
   D Dermanyssus

11. The stage in the life cycle of arachnids which has only has three pairs of legs is the

   A Nymph
   B Larva
   C Adult
   D Pupa

12. An individual segment of a tapeworm is a

   A Strobila
   B Scolex
   C Rostellum
   D Proglottid

13. Which tapeworm forms a hydatid cyst as its intermediate stage?

   A Taenia hydatigena
   B Taenia multiceps
   C Echinococcus granulosus
   D Dipylidium caninum

14. The drug that is effective against all tapeworms is

   A Fenbendazole
   B Praziquantel
   C Piperazine
   D Mebendazole

15. **Which statement is least accurate about the life cycle of Toxocara canis?**

    A The larvae can infest pups by two routes - via the mother's milk or by ingestion of infective eggs
    B It can be spread via paratenic hosts
    C Many cases of visceral larval migrans result in no clinical signs
    D Eggs that are passed in faeces take about 14 days to be infective

16. **What percentage of adult dogs have a patent infestation of Toxocara canis?**

    A 50%
    B 40%
    C 20%
    D 10%

17. **How can the eggs of Toxocara canis and Toxascaris leonina be differentiated from each other?**

    A The egg of Toxocara is much larger than that of Toxascaris
    B Toxascaris has a distinctive lemon-shaped egg
    C Toxocara has a rough, pitted shell
    D Toxascaris eggs are not found in faeces, since the larvae have already hatched and are present in the free larval form

18. **Of the following, which is the hookworm more commonly seen in dogs in the UK?**

    A Trichuris vulpis
    B Toxascaris leonina
    C Uncinaria stenocephala
    D Ancylostoma caninum

19. **What is the proper name of the heartworm?**

    A Dirofilaria immitis
    B Aelurostrongylus abstrusus
    C Capillaria plica
    D Toxoplasma gondii

20. **If a woman is infested with this parasite for the first time during her pregnancy, it could cause abortion. For which parasite is this statement true?**

    A   Toxocara canis
    B   Toxoplasma gondii
    C   Giardia
    D   Cryptosporidium

The answers are on page 237

13 General nursing

9 Questions

1. **Which formula should be used to determine daily basal energy requirements for patients over 5 kg?**

   A   BER (kcal) = 70 x bodyweight (in kg) + 30
   B   BER (kcal) = 30 x bodyweight (in kg) ÷ 70
   C   BER (kcal) = 30 x bodyweight (in kg) + 70
   D   BER (kcal) = 60 x bodyweight (in kg)

2. **The form of tube feeding that requires the use of an endoscope for its placement is**

   A   PEG tube
   B   Oesophagostomy tube
   C   Naso-oesophageal tube
   D   Enterostomy tube

3. **Which statement is true about the care of an older canine patient?**

   A   Higher protein levels are required in the diet, since many older animals have protein-losing diseases
   B   Exercise should be restricted to just one long walk per day
   C   Water should be freely available
   D   Changes in routine are not a problem, since mental ability is not usually affected

4. **The animal least at risk from the development of aspiration pneumonia is**

   A   An animal being syringe fed with the head tilted upwards
   B   An animal with megaoesophagus
   C   An animal recovering from an anaesthetic which still had food in its stomach
   D   A conscious animal that is vomiting

5. **If you were involved in the care of a paraplegic dog, which of the following would not be appropriate in its management?**

    A Provide a large kennel so that it is able to attempt to walk itself
    B Ensure that the animal has plenty of padding to lie on
    C Take the animal outside to stimulate urination and defaecation
    D Ensure that food and water are within reach of the patient

6. **Hypostatic pneumonia can be life threatening due to secondary infections. Which of the following methods is recommended to avoid this?**

    A Turn the patient twice daily
    B The patient should always remain in lateral recumbency
    C Coupage can be used 4-5 times daily
    D None of the above are appropriate management

7. **Which catheter is most suitable for use as an indwelling catheter in the bitch?**

    A Tieman's catheter
    B Foley catheter
    C Jackson catheter
    D Metal bitch catheter

8. **Petroleum jelly should not be used as a lubricant with which of the following catheters?**

    A Latex Foley catheter
    B Jackson cat catheter
    C Silicone Foley catheter
    D Teflon tomcat catheter

9. **Decubitus ulcers can be dressed with**

    A Barrier cream
    B Surgical spirit
    C Hydrogen peroxide
    D Dettol (chloroxylenol)

The answers are on page 243

14 Medical disorders and their nursing

35 Questions

Infectious diseases

1. **Which of the following statements is untrue?**

   A A vector is another animal which carries the organism
   B The intermediate hosts of tapeworms are a form of vector
   C A fomite is an inanimate object which can act as the means by which an organism may be passed between one animal and another e.g. food bowl
   D Vertical transmission refers to transmission from a young animal to its sibling

2. **The disease that can be described as infectious but not contagious is**

   A Sarcoptic mange
   B Parvovirus
   C Pyometra
   D Diabetes mellitus

3. **An animal that has never been ill and is healthy, but is shedding organism, is called a**

   A Healthy carrier
   B Convalescent carrier
   C Closed carrier
   D Clinically affected carrier

4. **The canine infectious disease which can lead to animals developing encephalitis in older age is**

   A Parvovirus
   B Infectious canine hepatitis
   C Lyme disease
   D Canine distemper

5. **If parvovirus affects young pups from an unvaccinated bitch, what signs may be seen?**

   A Painful abdomen and petechial haemorrhages
   B Jaundice
   C Cardiac failure
   D Respiratory signs

6. **The causal agent of infectious canine hepatitis is**

   A Bordetella bronchiseptica
   B Canine adenovirus 1
   C Borrelia burgdorferi
   D Leptospira icterohaemorrhagiae

7. **The complication that may result after apparent recovery from canine adenovirus 1 infection is**

   A Corneal oedema
   B Stunting and discolouration of the teeth
   C Permanent malabsorption problems
   D Chronic liver failure

8. **Of the following, which canine infectious organism is potentially zoonotic?**

   A Canine adenovirus 1
   B Leptospira canicola
   C Distemper virus
   D Canine parainfluenza virus

9. **The disease caused by a bacterium is**

   A Lyme disease
   B Infectious canine hepatitis
   C Distemper
   D Rabies

10. **Which canine infectious disease can lead to the development of respiratory signs?**

    A Parvovirus
    B Infectious canine hepatitis
    C Distemper
    D Leptospirosis

11. **Of the feline infectious diseases, which of the following usually leads to severe conjunctivitis and chemosis, and occasionally to abortion in the pregnant queen?**

    A Feline leukaemia virus
    B Feline panleucopaenia
    C Feline infectious anaemia
    D Chlamydia psittaci

12. **Many infectious diseases can be prevented through judicious use of vaccination. However, which of the feline diseases cannot be vaccinated against in the UK?**

    A Feline leukaemia virus
    B Chlamydia psittaci
    C Feline infectious peritonitis
    D Feline herpes virus

13. **The most common FeLV associated disease is**

    A Lymphosarcoma
    B Feline infectious anaemia
    C Immune-mediated haemolytic anaemia
    D Abortion

14. **Which cats are most likely to become persistently infected with FeLV?**

    A Kittens infected in utero
    B Kittens infected that are less than 8 weeks of age
    C Cats between the ages of 1 and 8 years
    D Cats over the age of 8 years

15. **In which feline disease do antibody-antigen complexes cause a vasculitis which results in the production of a fluid exudate within the thoracic or abdominal cavity?**

    A Feline infectious anaemia
    B Feline infectious peritonitis
    C Feline infectious enteritis
    D Feline immunodeficiency virus

16. **If an animal tests positive for FIV but is clinically well, what advice should be given to the owner?**

    A The cat should be euthanased immediately
    B The cat should be retested in 12 weeks; many cats recover
    C The cat should be kept indoors, away from other cats, until it falls ill, when it may require euthanasia
    D No particular precautions need to be taken, since transfer to other cats is rare

17. **Which organism does not show latency?**

    A Haemobartonella felis
    B Feline leukaemia virus
    C Feline herpes virus
    D Feline calici virus

18. **Which canine disease is closely related to feline panleucopaenia?**

    A Canine parvovirus
    B Canine distemper
    C Canine infectious hepatitis
    D Lyme disease

Non-infectious diseases

19. **Which of the following methods of giving oxygen could lead to hyperthermia if an animal is panting excessively?**

    A Mask
    B Flow by
    C Buster collar and cling film
    D Nasal tube

20. **An animal with laryngeal paralysis would show which of the following signs?**

    A Exercise intolerance
    B A change in bark
    C Respiratory stertor
    D All of the above

21. **All of the following heart diseases are congenital except**

    A Patent ductus arteriosus
    B Endocardiosis
    C Ventricular septal defect
    D Tetralogy of Fallot

22. **Why is nitroglycerine ointment used in the management of a case with acute heart failure?**

    A It is a diuretic, and acts to reduce the load on the heart by reducing circulating blood volume
    B It improves the oxygen carrying capacity of the blood, thereby improving oxygenation of the tissues
    C It increases the heart muscle's force of contraction
    D It is a venodilator, and reduces the workload of the heart by lowering blood pressure

23. **Which of the following problems does not lead to anaemia?**

    A Iron deficiency
    B Polycythaemia
    C Chronic renal failure
    D Von Willebrand's disease

24. **An animal showing pharyngeal retching, regurgitation or vomiting can all be described by the owner as it being sick. It is important to identify more specifically which process is actually occurring. Which description below most closely describes vomiting?**

   A The animal gags and retches and usually brings up a small amount of mucus and phlegm. This may come down the nose

   B The animal usually starts to salivate, and then abdominal contractions start before the animal brings up partially digested food

   C The animal lowers its head, and undigested food is brought up. This usually happens 10-15 minutes after eating

   D Vomiting is different from any of the descriptions given

25. **Which of the following problems would not lead to an animal developing diarrhoea?**

   A Exocrine pancreatic insufficiency

   B Inflammatory bowel disease

   C Worm infestation

   D Key-Gaskell syndrome (feline dysautonomia)

26. **The owner of a dog which has just started vomiting, but is bright in itself, calls for advice. Which is least appropriate?**

   A There is no need to do anything; most cases resolve spontaneously

   B Starve the animal for 24 hours, giving just small amounts of water

   C After starvation, start small easily digestible meals

   D If there is no improvement after starvation, or if the animal deteriorates in condition, then it should be seen by a veterinary surgeon

27. **Which clinical sign is more indicative of diarrhoea due to large intestinal problems rather than small intestinal?**

   A The animal is hungry, but shows weight loss

   B The animal passes faeces very frequently, often with blood and mucus

   C Borborygmi is common

   D There is no tenesmus when faeces are passed

28. **Acute renal failure can be caused in three different ways - pre-renal causes, renal causes or post-renal causes. Which of the following is a post-renal cause?**

    A Dehydration
    B Shock
    C Bladder rupture
    D Ethylene glycol toxicity

29. **Which disease can be tested for using a low dose dexamethasone screening test?**

    A Hyperadrenocorticism
    B Hyperthyroidism
    C Hyperparathyroidism
    D Hyperinsulinaemia

30. **The clinical signs associated with hyperparathyroidism are**

    A Bilateral symmetrical alopecia
    B Increased appetite but weight loss
    C Hypocalcaemia, muscle spasm and rigidity
    D Reduced bone density and spontaneous fractures

31. **Which term relates to an animal that is paralysed on one side of the body, but not the other?**

    A Paraplegia
    B Hemiplegia
    C Quadriplegia
    D Tetrapelgia

32. **The bone disease that develops as a result of intra-thoracic or intra-abdominal masses is**

    A Rickets
    B Metaphyseal osteopathy
    C Osteochondrosis
    D Hypertrophic osteodystrophy

33. **Which reproductive hormone, if present in large amounts, can lead to bone marrow suppression?**

    A Testosterone
    B Progesterone
    C Oestrogen
    D Luteinising hormone

34. **An acute allergic reaction in which an animal develops multiple small pruritic swellings in the skin is described as**

    A Impetigo
    B Furunculosis
    C Atopic dermatitis
    D Urticaria

35. **Intradermal skin testing is used to test for which type of allergic disease?**

    A Dietary hypersensitivity
    B Contact dermatitis
    C Atopic dermatitis
    D Urticaria

The answers are on page 247

15 Obstetric and paediatric nursing of the dog and cat

18 Questions

1. **Under which piece of legislation do owners have a responsibility to ensure that pups or kitten sold are clinically healthy and have a sound temperament?**

    A Trade Description Act
    B Breeding and Sale of Dogs (Welfare) Act 1999
    C Sale of Goods Act
    D Protection of Animals Acts

2. **By when should the testes have descended in a male dog?**

    A Birth
    B 5 days after birth
    C 10 days after birth
    D 1 month after birth

3. **Which term is used to describe the retention of a testis (or both testes) in the abdomen?**

    A Anorchia
    B Cryptorchidism
    C Monorchidism
    D Orchitis

4. **The fraction of the canine ejaculate that contains the sperm is the**

   A First fraction
   B Second fraction
   C Third fraction
   D All the fractions contain sperm, but in varying quantities

5. **Under normal circumstances, how long is metoestrus in the bitch?**

   A 7 days
   B 4 months
   C 7 months
   D 55 days

6. **The statement about the reproductive cycle of the queen that is correct is**

   A She is a spontaneous ovulator and a non-seasonal breeder
   B She is an induced ovulator and a non-seasonal breeder
   C She is a spontaneous ovulator and a seasonal breeder
   D She is an induced ovulator and a seasonal breeder

7. **Blood tests can be used to determine whether a bitch is in oestrus or not. Which hormone's presence is tested for?**

   A Progesterone
   B Oestrogen
   C Luteinising hormone
   D Follicle-stimulating hormone

8. **Occasionally animals are born which have both male and female genital tissue. Which statement about these animals is true?**

   A They are true hermaphrodites and can self fertilise
   B They should be described as intersexes
   C Only the male genitals will function, though they have a small uterus
   D The animal will have functional ovaries

9. **Of the following methods of pregnancy diagnosis, which can be used earliest in the bitch?**

   A Abdominal palpation
   B Identification of foetal heart beats
   C Radiography
   D Ultrasound

10. **Which definition is incorrect?**

    A The term foetus can be used to describe the developing young from day 10 after ovulation
    B Resorption is the complete reabsorption of the zygote occurring early in pregnancy
    C Abortion occurs when a dead foetus is expelled before day 58 of pregnancy
    D Stillbirth is the delivery of a dead foetus after day 58 of pregnancy

11. **The temperature of the area where the bitch is due to whelp should be maintained at**

    A 15-20°C
    B 20-25°C
    C 25-30°C
    D 30-35°C

12. **Of the following, which is not a sign of imminent parturition?**

    A A rise in body temperature of about 2°C
    B Nesting behaviour
    C Intermittent contractions
    D Shivering and restlessness

13. **Dystocia can be described as foetal or maternal dystocia, dependent on cause. Which of these would be a foetal dystocia?**

    A Uterine inertia
    B Obstructive dystocia
    C Exhaustion
    D Breech birth

14. **From what age would you expect a pup to be able to stand?**

    A   2 days
    B   5 days
    C   10 days
    D   3 weeks

15. **How long does the puerperium last?**

    A   2 weeks
    B   3 weeks
    C   4 weeks
    D   6 weeks

16. **Placental retention might be identifiable clinically by**

    A   An increase in the dam's temperature without any other signs
    B   A persistent green vulval discharge
    C   Swelling and hardness of the mammary glands
    D   Rejection of the young by the mother

17. **A dam normally needs to stimulate urination and defaecation in neonatal pups or kittens. For how long after birth does she need to do this?**

    A   2 days
    B   5 days
    C   1-2 weeks
    D   2-3 weeks

18. **Which congenital deformity poses no threat to the animal's health?**

    A   Atresia ani
    B   Polydactyly
    C   Open fontanelle
    D   Cleft palate

The answers are on page 260

16 Surgical and high-dependence nursing

36 Questions

1. **Of the following, which is not a cardinal sign of inflammation?**

   A Redness
   B Heat
   C Loss of function
   D Pus

2. **The fluid formed as a result of inflammation that contains white cells and proteinaceous debris is**

   A Transudate
   B Modified transudate
   C Exudate
   D Chyle

3. **Surgical removal of the gall bladder is termed a**

   A Celiotomy
   B Cholecystectomy
   C Orchidectomy
   D Tenotomy

4. **For how long can a fresh open wound be considered contaminated but not infected?**

   A 6 hours
   B 10 hours
   C 14 hours
   D 24 hours

5. **The clipper blade that should be used for an animal's final clip prior to surgery is a**

   A   No. 10 blade
   B   No. 20 blade
   C   No. 30 blade
   D   No. 40 blade

6. **As a guideline, what minimum margin from the incision site should be clipped and prepped prior to surgery?**

   A   5 cm
   B   10 cm
   C   15 cm
   D   20 cm

7. **Post-operative bandages be always checked and changed. How long after application should this take place?**

   A   12 hours
   B   24 hours
   C   48 hours
   D   72 hours

8. **Which solution is suitable for lavage of a contaminated wound?**

   A   0.5% chlorhexidine solution
   B   1% hydrogen peroxide solution
   C   Cetrimide/cetavlon solution (Savlon)
   D   Hypochlorite solution

9. **The types of primary dressing material that stimulate the production of granulation tissue and can be used to control low level haemorrhage are**

   A   Saline-soaked gauze swabs
   B   Non-adherent paraffin gauze dressings
   C   Alginate dressings
   D   Hydrogel dressings

10. **Free skin grafts may fail for a number of reasons. Which is not a reason this could occur?**

    A Inadequate preparation of the wound bed
    B The graft was not immobilised properly
    C The dressing and bandage was left on for 5-7 days
    D Serum or haemorrhage accumulated under the graft

11. **Of the following topical wound treatments, which actively stimulates the development of granulation tissue?**

    A Aloe vera ointment
    B Malic, benzoic and salicylic acid solution
    C Zinc bacitracin ointment
    D Silver sulphadiazine ointment

12. **External coaption techniques can be used on some types of fractures. Which fracture could be treated this way?**

    A Mid-shaft femoral fracture
    B Scapular fracture
    C Transverse fracture of the radius and ulna
    D Spiral fracture of the tibia

13. **The statement that is untrue about the advantages of internal fixation techniques for fractures is**

    A The limb can return to full function earlier than with other repair techniques
    B Internal fixation is only suitable for some types of fractures
    C The reduction is more accurate than with other repair methods
    D Fractures in any location can be managed

14. **Which type of plate is parallel sided with between 4 and 8 round screw holes?**

    A Sherman plate
    B Dynamic compression plate
    C Venables plate
    D Lane plate

15. **After external coaption methods have been used for stabilisation of a fracture, it is possible for complications to develop. Which statement about these is true?**

    A Osteomyelitis is common
    B Fracture disease may develop
    C Pressure sores are rarely a problem
    D The implant may stimulate an immune reaction

16. **What is an allograft?**

    A A skin graft harvested from another animal
    B A bone graft taken from the same animal, but a different bone
    C A skin graft taken from the same animal, but a different location
    D A bone graft taken from a different animal, but of the same species

17. **Luxation of which joint is most commonly the result of congenital problems?**

    A Hip
    B Patella
    C Elbow
    D Carpus

18. **Which tumour with the word ending usually reserved for benign tumours is actually very often malignant?**

    A Papilloma
    B Fibroma
    C Lipoma
    D Melanoma

19. **Of the following statements about tumours, which is true?**

    A Sarcomas are malignant tumours of connective tissue
    B Carcinomas are benign tumours of epithelial tissue
    C Adenomas are benign tumours formed from fatty tissue
    D Fibrosarcomas are found exclusively in the skin

20. **Clean-contaminated could be used to described which of these procedures?**

    A Umbilical hernia repair
    B Oral surgery
    C Gastrotomy
    D Closure of a recent traumatic wound (less than 4 hours old)

21. **The term keratitis describes which of the following?**

    A Inflammation of the skin
    B Overflow of tears
    C Inflammation of the cornea
    D Inflammation of the eyelids

22. **Left untreated, which ocular condition will lead to permanent damage to the retina and blindness?**

    A Glaucoma
    B Distichiasis
    C Cataract formation
    D Corneal foreign body

23. **Which statement about mammary tumours is incorrect?**

    A The surgical removal of a single affected gland is called a mammmectomy
    B Drains should be used after mammary gland surgery to prevent the formation of seromas
    C A radical mastectomy involves removal of all the mammary glands on one side of the body
    D Mammary tumours in the cat are usually benign

24. **The extraction of which type of tooth could result in the formation of an oronasal fistula?**

    A Incisor
    B Canine
    C Premolar
    D Molar

25. **The most appropriate solution to use as a mouthwash for animals is**

   A 2% hydrogen peroxide solution
   B 0.2% chlorhexidine solution
   C 2% povidone-iodine solution
   D 0.1% hypochlorite solution

26. **What is the minimum length of time a gastrostomy tube should be left in place?**

   A 24 hours
   B 48 hours
   C 5 days
   D 10 days

27. **Several breeds suffer from the brachycephalic airway obstruction syndrome (BAOS). Which of the following does not contribute to this syndrome?**

   A Stenotic nares
   B Hypoplastic trachea
   C Long soft palate
   D Bronchial inflammation

28. **Which clinical sign in a male dog is suggestive of a Sertoli cell tumour?**

   A Gynaecomastia
   B Increased libido
   C Lethargy and bradycardia
   D Development of anal adenomas

29. **A rupture in which the contents become devitalised due to compression of the blood vessels supplying them is described as**

   A Irreducible
   B Strangulated
   C Incarcerated
   D Reducible

30. **The operative procedure to surgically fuse a joint and prevent its movement is an**

    A Arthrodesis
    B Arthroscopy
    C Arthropexy
    D Arthrotomy

31. **Which of the following factors can contribute to the development of a nosocomial infection?**

    A Minimal staff being involved with each individual patient
    B Regular cleaning of kennels and surrounding areas
    C Treatments such as intravenous and urinary catheters
    D Treatment of infectious disease by appropriate antibiotics

32. **The least reactive material to be made into urinary catheters is**

    A Silicone
    B Polyvinyl chloride
    C Polypropylene
    D Polyethylene

33. **If a pulse oximeter is to be used during patient monitoring, above what level should oxygen saturation remain?**

    A Above 90%
    B Above 93%
    C Above 95%
    D Above 97%

34. **Which statement is true about the assessment of blood pressure?**

    A Palpation of peripheral pulses is a useful assessment of blood pressure
    B Oscillometric measurements of blood pressure are more accurate than the use of Doppler systems
    C Blood pressure can be measured by the placement of an arterial catheter connected to a manometer
    D Measurement of central venous pressure is based on pressure measurements taken from the cephalic vein

35. **All of the following are forms of physiotherapy. Which may be used to provide some pain relief?**

    A Contrast bathing
    B Efflurage
    C Petrissage
    D Transcutaneous electrical nerve stimulation (TENS)

36. **Total parenteral nutrition can be supplied by which of the following techniques?**

    A Feeding via a naso-gastric tube
    B Feeding via a PEG tube
    C Feeding via an intravenous line
    D Feeding via an oesophagostomy tube

The answers are on page 265

17 Theatre practice

21 Questions

1. **Which statement about sterilisation and disinfection is true?**

   A Asepsis is the absence of micro-organisms and spores
   B Disinfection is the destruction of all micro-organisms and spores
   C Sterilisation can only be achieved by the use of heat in the form of dry heat or steam
   D Antisepsis is the removal of all micro-organisms and spores from the environment

2. **Of the following procedures, which would be classed as contaminated?**

   A Repair of a closed fracture that occurred two days previously
   B Debriding an infected bite wound
   C Gastrotomy to remove a foreign body
   D Repair of a fresh wound to the thigh region

3. **What colour does the fluid in Browne's tube change from and to during the sterilisation process?**

   A Green to blue
   B Blue to clear
   C Red to green
   D Yellow to red

4. **Sterilisation of instruments in a hot air oven operating at 150°C takes**

   A 30 minutes
   B 60 minutes
   C 120 minutes
   D 180 minutes

5. **For an ideal operating theatre, which of the following is untrue?**

A There should be a swing door into theatre which is normally kept closed

B Open shelves are the best means for storing equipment in theatre

C Good lighting is essential - both an ambient light source and an adjustable directional surgical light should be present

D Windows should not open

6. **How frequently should surgical masks be changed if being worn in theatre?**

A Daily

B Every 2 hours

C Between every procedure

D Hourly

7. **There are advantages and disadvantages with clipping the fur prior to anaesthesia. Which of the following statements is untrue?**

A Clipping under anaesthesia decreases asepsis

B Clipping over 12 hours before surgery reduces the number of skin bacteria

C Two or more people are always required if the patient is not anaesthetised

D Clipping prior to anaesthesia means that the period of anaesthesia is shorter

8. **Esmarch's bandage is used to**

A Support the hindlimb after reduction of a luxated hip

B Support the forelimb after shoulder surgery

C Hold dressings in place over a gastrostomy site

D Create a bloodless surgical field which is maintained by the use of a tourniquet

9. **Of the following statements regarding the cleaning of surgical instruments, which is true?**

   A Instruments should be cleaned with a brush under very hot water
   B All ratchets and box joints should be closed before submerging in an ultrasonic cleaner
   C Instrument cleaning solutions containing enzymes may be used
   D Debris on hard to clean areas should be removed with an abrasive powder

10. **The scalpel blade with a fine straight cutting edge, sometimes referred to as a tenotomy blade, is**

    A Size 10
    B Size 11
    C Size 12
    D Size 15

11. **Sutures can be removed post-operatively using which type of scissors?**

    A Pains scissors
    B Carless scissors
    C Mayo scissors
    D Metzenbaum scissors

12. **There are several retractors designed to hold back tissues during surgery. Which would be suitable for use during abdominal surgery to hold back the abdominal wall?**

    A Travers retractor
    B Balfour retractor
    C West's retractor
    D Gelpi retractor

13. **ASIF equipment is different from other types of orthopaedic equipment. Which statement is true about this?**

    A It is more highly engineered, meaning that it offers the ability to repair fractures with greater precision
    B It is less expensive than other orthopaedic equipment, making its use more popular
    C The drill and screw sizes are all in imperial measurements
    D The most commonly used bone plate from the ASIF range is the Venables plate

14. **The method of sterilisation most suitable for a fibre-optic flexible endoscope would be**

    A Autoclave
    B Hot air oven
    C Alcohol
    D Ethylene oxide

15. **The tendency of a suture material to coil back into its original packaged shape is described as**

    A Drag
    B Capillarity
    C Chatter
    D Memory

16. **Of the following suture materials, which is non-absorbable?**

    A Polyglycolic acid
    B Polyamide
    C Polyglyconate
    D Polydioxanone

17. **The suture material removed from the operation site by phagocytosis is**

    A Catgut
    B Polyglactin 910
    C Polyesters
    D Linen

18. **The continuous suture pattern suitable for skin closure is**

    A Ford interlocking
    B Simple interrupted
    C Cruciate mattress
    D Horizontal mattress

19. **Of the following sized suture materials, which is the smallest?**

    A 2/0
    B 3 metric
    C 6/0
    D 6 metric

20. **The forceps used for laying out an instrument trolley are**

    A Rampley's forceps
    B Cheatle forceps
    C Rochester-Pean forceps
    D Crile's forceps

21. **A laparotomy incision made parallel to, but to one side of, the linea alba can be described as**

    A Paramedian
    B Paracostal
    C Sublumbar
    D Midline

The answers are on page 276

18 Fluid therapy and shock

15 Questions

1. **A small water-soluble particle carrying one or more positive charges is called a/an**

   A Anion
   B Cation
   C Electrolyte
   D Ion

2. **The main intracellular anions are**

   A Chloride and bicarbonate
   B Sodium and calcium
   C Chloride and phosphate
   D Phosphate and protein

3. **How much of a healthy animal's water requirement is generated through metabolic processes?**

   A About 5%
   B About 10%
   C About 30%
   D About 50%

4. **Urine specific gravity measurement can be used to provide an indication of how concentrated a sample is. Which of the following is within the isosthenuric range?**

   A 1.006
   B 1.010
   C 1.030
   D 1.080

5. **What is the estimated fluid deficit for a 20 kg dog with a PCV of 50%?**

   A 50 ml
   B 500 ml
   C 1000 ml
   D 2000 ml

6. **Metabolic acidosis could be caused by which of the following conditions?**

   A Chronic renal failure
   B Prepyloric vomiting
   C Lung damage
   D Hyperventilation

7. **An over-the-needle catheter should be replaced every**

   A 12 hours
   B 24 hours
   C 48 hours
   D 96 hours

8. **The most suitable route for fluid therapy for a severely dehydrated puppy would be**

   A Subcutaneous administration
   B Intraperitoneal administration
   C Rectal administration
   D Intraosseous administration

9. **When collecting blood for transfusion, the usual anticoagulant is**

   A Lithium heparin
   B Sodium citrate
   C Acid citrate dextrose
   D Fluoride-oxalate

10. **Which of the following solutions is hypertonic?**

   A Gelatin solution
   B Dextran solution
   C Hartmann's solution
   D 0.9% saline

11. **It is unsafe to add sodium bicarbonate to Hartmann's or Ringer's solution. What is the reason for this?**

    A It makes the solution too hypertonic; it will dehydrate the animal's cells
    B It reacts with calcium to form a solid precipitate
    C It means that the animal would be overdosed with sodium
    D Potassium and bicarbonate are incompatible

12. **An animal which was becoming overhydrated would not show which of the following signs?**

    A Respiratory distress
    B Chemosis
    C Nasal discharge
    D Oliguria

13. **The clinical sign not usually seen in shock is**

    A Tachycardia
    B Hypothermia
    C Oliguria
    D Hypertension

14. **Which fluid would be appropriate to use to maintain an anorexic cat which had not become significantly dehydrated yet?**

    A Hartmann's solution
    B 0.18% saline + 4% dextrose
    C 5% dextrose
    D Ringer's solution

15. **Calculate the initial drip rate for an animal that is 2880 ml dehydrated, assuming that you wish to give half the fluid deficit in the first 6 hours, and that 1 ml contains 15 drops**

    A 2 drops per second
    B 1 drop per second
    C 1 drop every 2 seconds
    D 4 drops every 3 seconds

The answers are on page 282

19 Anaesthesia and analgesia

30 Questions

1. Pre-operative assessment is an important part of the anaesthetic protocol. Which of the following statements about pre-operative assessment is untrue?

   A Liver disease would tend to cause a patient to remain unconscious for longer than normal
   B Cases showing renal dysfunction should be supported by intravenous fluids throughout anaesthesia
   C Older animals are always at greater risk than young patients
   D Epileptic animals on treatment may be more resistant to anaesthetic agents than normal patients

2. Which of the following drugs is an alpha-2 agonist?

   A Xylazine
   B Atipamezole
   C Diazepam
   D Acepromazine

3. Of the following drugs, which has no analgesic effect?

   A Buprenorphine
   B Acepromazine
   C Medetomidine
   D Lignocaine

4. **Which commonly used opiate has the longest duration of action?**

   A Morphine
   B Pethidine
   C Butorphanol
   D Buprenorphine

5. **Which group of drugs may cause gastric irritation?**

   A Opiates
   B Alpha-2 agonists
   C Anticholinergics
   D Non-steroidal anti-inflammatories

6. **Adrenaline is often added to local anaesthetic preparations. What effect does this have?**

   A It increases the potency of the nerve block
   B It increases the recovery from the nerve block
   C It increases the duration of the nerve block
   D It increases the pH of the area and improves penetration of the tissue by the anaesthetic

7. **What is the concentration in mg/ml of a 5% solution?**

   A 0.5 mg/ml
   B 50 mg/ml
   C 0.2 mg/ml
   D 5 mg/ml

8. **Local anaesthetics can be used in a number of ways. Which method of use is defined as drug injection in the proximity of identifiable nerves?**

   A Surface block
   B Epidural block
   C Perineural block
   D IVRA

9. **Which drug, if injected perivascularly, may cause tissue necrosis?**

   A   Thiopentone
   B   Propofol
   C   Ketamine
   D   Alphaxalone and alphadolone

10. **The anaesthetic agent Saffan is which of the following types of drug?**

   A   A barbiturate
   B   A steroid
   C   A dissociative anaesthetic
   D   A phenol

11. **Inhalation anaesthetic agents can be described by MAC numbers. What information does this provide about the drug?**

   A   The potency of the drug
   B   The solubility of the drug in the bloodstream
   C   The rate of recovery from the drug
   D   The way in which the drug is removed from the body

12. **Which inhalation agent degrades in the presence of soda-lime?**

   A   Ether
   B   Sevoflurane
   C   Isoflurane
   D   Halothane

13. **The least potent inhalation agent is**

   A   Methoxyflurane
   B   Sevoflurane
   C   Nitrous oxide
   D   Isoflurane

14. Which statement about anaesthetic gas scavenging is untrue?

A Canister scavengers are not effective at removing nitrous oxide from exhaled gases
B Passive scavenging requires the use of a fan
C Canister scavengers should be weighed to determine when they are exhausted
D The maximum acceptable length of tubing for passive scavenging is 2.6 m (8 feet)

15. The normal ratio of nitrous oxide to oxygen used in inhalation anaesthesia is

A 1:2
B 2:1
C 1:3
D 3:1

16. Of the following anaesthetic circuits, which is not good for intermittent positive pressure ventilation (IPPV)?

A Ayre's T-piece with Jackson-Rees modification
B To and Fro
C Bain
D Magill

17. What figure may be used as an estimate of an animal's minute volume in order to calculate the fresh gas flow rate?

A 20 ml/kg/min
B 30 ml/kg/min
C 200 ml/kg/min
D 1 litre/kg/min

18. The circuit factor for a Lack circuit is

A 1 - 1.5
B 2 - 2.5
C 2.5 - 3
D 3 - 3.5

19. **Small portable anaesthetic machines usually use which sized gas cylinders?**

    A A
    B B
    C D
    D E

20. **The gas is contained in grey cylinders is**

    A Oxygen
    B Carbon dioxide
    C Cyclopropane
    D Nitrous oxide

21. **Neuro-muscular blockers can be used to facilitate a number of surgical procedures. Which statement is untrue about these drugs?**

    A Gallamine is the most commonly used neuro-muscular blocker
    B Succinyl choline is a depolarising blocker
    C Atracurium spontaneously breaks down in the body and does not require metabolism
    D Neuro-muscular blockers may be used to facilitate IPPV

22. **Other than neostigmine, which drug can be used to antagonise neuro-muscular blockade?**

    A Naloxone .
    B Atipamezole
    C Diprenorphine
    D Edrophonium

23. **The stage of anaesthesia that is the stage of voluntary excitement is**

    A Stage I
    B Stage II
    C Stage III
    D Stage IV

24. **If mucous membranes appear *bright* pink whilst an animal is under anaesthesia, what might this suggest?**

   A Good tissue oxygenation
   B Shock
   C Hypercapnia
   D Poor peripheral perfusion

25. **Which of the following drugs would be metabolised most slowly?**

   A Thiopentone sodium
   B Alphaxalone and alphadolone
   C Propofol
   D Methohexitone sodium

26. **Which description best describes the Magill circuit?**

   A There is a single piece of tubing connecting the anaesthetic machine and animal, with a valve close to the animal and a reservoir bag close to the machine
   B There is a single piece of tubing connecting the anaesthetic machine and animal, with a valve close to the machine and a reservoir bag close to the animal
   C There is a single piece of tubing connecting the anaesthetic machine and animal, with both the valve and a reservoir bag close to the machine
   D There is a single piece of tubing connecting the anaesthetic machine and animal, with both the valve and a reservoir bag close to the animal

27. **Which is not a recommended procedure for ensuring that exposure to inhalation agents by staff is minimised?**

   A Patients should be intubated, and the cuff inflated
   B The vaporiser should only be turned on after the patient has been connected to the circuit
   C Pure oxygen should be given for at least 30 seconds prior to disconnecting
   D Vaporisers should be filled at the start of the operating session

28. **If needing to anaesthetise a neonate, which statement is true about special considerations that should be made?**

A Oxygen consumption is lower than that of an adult
B Hypotension is less likely in the neonate than an older animal
C Neonates should not be starved for longer than 2-3 hours
D Drug dosages per kilogram bodyweight are usually more than for an adult of the same species

29. **Surgery on which part of the body may lead to a reflex slowing of the heart rate?**

A Kidney
B Eye
C Uterus
D Thyroid

30. **Which drug in an anaesthetic emergency box may be used in cases of hypotension?**

A Bicarbonate
B Lignocaine
C Atropine
D Dobutamine

The answers are on page 286

20 Diagnostic imaging

24 Questions

1. **Which statement about the electromagnetic spectrum is true?**

   A   All waves on the spectrum have the same frequency
   B   α and β particles are also found on the spectrum as well as X-rays and γ-rays
   C   Waves with high frequency also have long wavelength
   D   All waves on the electromagnetic spectrum travel at the same speed

2. **The function of the aluminium filter across the window of the X-ray tube head is**

   A   To focus the X-ray beam onto the item to be radiographed
   B   To absorb 'soft' or low-powered X-rays which would not be diagnostic, just harmful to the patient
   C   To absorb heat generated as X-rays pass through
   D   To prevent X-rays being scattered

3. **What is the purpose of the oil bath which surrounds the glass envelope of the tube head?**

   A   It acts to lubricate the movement of the tube head within its metal casing
   B   It absorbs X-rays travelling in directions other than that required for radiography
   C   It acts as a heat sink, for the heat generated in the target area of the tube head
   D   It acts as an insulator and prevents cooling of the tube head in cold conditions

4. **There are three important controls that are altered to adjust X-ray exposures. Which statement is untrue about these?**

   A mA controls the number of X-rays produced
   B kV controls the penetrating power or quality of the X-ray beam
   C The timer determines how long the kV is applied for
   D The mA control alters the potential difference between the cathode and the anode of the X-ray tube head

5. **When making an exposure, how far away from the primary beam should an operator be?**

   A At least 1 metre
   B At least 2 metres
   C At least 3 metres
   D At least 4 metres

6. **If an exposure was taken and the kV was too high, how would the radiograph appear?**

   A The tissues would be overpenetrated, and the whole radiograph would be dark
   B The tissues would be underpenetrated, so the image would be pale with a black background
   C The radiograph would be pale with a pale background
   D None of the above would take place

7. **Which formula for calculating a new mAs is correct when altering the focal-film distance?**

   A $\text{New mAs} = \text{Old mAs}^2 \times \dfrac{\text{New distance}}{\text{Old distance}}$

   B $\text{New mAs} = \text{Old mAs} \times \dfrac{\text{Old distance}^2}{\text{New distance}^2}$

   C $\text{New mAs} = \text{New distance} \times \dfrac{\text{Old distance}^2}{\text{Old mAs}}$

   D $\text{New mAs} = \text{Old mAs} \times \dfrac{\text{New distance}^2}{\text{Old distance}^2}$

8. **Scattered radiation is hazardous to both patient and operator. Which of the following would not reduce the amount of scattered radiation produced?**

   A Reduction of the kV
   B Use of a grid
   C Collimation of the primary beam
   D Use of a lead top on the table

9. **The type of grid most effective at avoiding grid cut off is**

   A Parallel grid
   B Focused grid
   C Pseudo-focused grid
   D Crossed parallel grid

10. **Which layer of the X-ray film contains the X-ray sensitive grains of silver bromide?**

    A Polyester base
    B Subbing layer
    C Emulsion
    D Supercoat

11. **X-ray film is used for a number of different purposes, and therefore is available in various forms and speeds. Which requires the highest exposures?**

    A Fast screen film
    B Slow screen film
    C Mammography film
    D Non-screen film

12. **The active chemical in the developer is**

    A Phenidone hydroquinone
    B Ammonium thiosulphate
    C Sodium thiosulphate
    D Silver halide

13. **For manual processing, at what temperature is the developer tank usually kept?**

    A   10°C
    B   15°C
    C   20°C
    D   25°C

14. **What is meant by the somatic effects of X-rays?**

    A   Changes in tissues such as damage to the intestinal wall leading to vomiting and dehydration
    B   Induction of neoplastic growths in tissues exposed to radiation
    C   Damage to the sperm or ova
    D   All of the above

15. **The minimum thickness of lead equivalence required for a lead apron is**

    A   0.1 mm
    B   0.25 mm
    C   0.35 mm
    D   0.5 mm

16. **Barium sulphate is a commonly used contrast medium. Which statement is untrue about its use?**

    A   It can be used mixed with food in the form of a paste to highlight the oesophagus
    B   It can be administered as an enema to highlight the colon
    C   It must not be used in cases where perforation is suspected
    D   It can be used in the respiratory tract to highlight the trachea and bronchi

17. **The technique used to highlight the ureters is**

    A   Pneumocystography
    B   Intravenous urography
    C   Retrograde urethrography
    D   Double contrast cystography

18. **Ultrasound waves are produced due to the**

    A Photo-electric effect
    B Compton effect
    C Piezo-electric effect
    D Thermionic emission

19. **A screening scheme using ultrasonography has been set up for which of the following diseases in cats?**

    A Polycystic kidney disease
    B Cholangiohepatitis
    C Ectopic ureters
    D Megacolon

20. **Which of the following imaging techniques uses radioactive substances which are injected into the patient and a gamma camera?**

    A Computed tomography
    B Magnetic Resonance Imaging (MRI)
    C Scintigraphy
    D Ultrasonography

21. **During which stage of processing is unexposed silver halide removed from the X-ray film?**

    A Washing
    B Development
    C Fixing
    D Drying

22. **Where should you centre the X-ray beam for a radiograph of the lateral thorax?**

    A Level with the last rib, midway between dorsal and ventral skin surfaces
    B Level with the caudal border of the scapula, midway between dorsal and ventral skin surfaces
    C On the thoracic inlet
    D On the thoraco-lumbar junction

23. **A radiograph is taken with the following exposure factors: 80 kV, 10 mA and 0.5 seconds. There is a lot of scattered radiation reaching the film, so you decide to decrease the kV by 10. Which of the following settings could you use?**

    A 70 kV, 20 mA, 0.5 seconds
    B 70 kV, 20 mA, 1 second
    C 80 kV, 20 mA, 0.5 seconds
    D 70 kV, 10 mA, 0.7 seconds

24. **If you are manually processing non-screen film at standard temperatures, how long should it be left in the developer?**

    A 3 minutes
    B 4 minutes
    C 5 minutes
    D 6 minutes

The answers are on page 293

Answers

1 Anatomy and physiology

Terminology and directional terms

1. D   **The term relating to structures closer to the trunk is proximal**

Cranial means towards the head.

Ventral means towards the underside of the animal.

Medial means towards the midline of the body.

2. D   **The under surface of the hind paw is described as plantar**

The same surface in the fore paw is described as palmar.

3. C   **The zygomatic arch is the most rostral structure listed**

The zygomatic arch is formed by the zygomatic bone and the temporal bone and is more commonly referred to as the 'cheekbone'. The term rostral is used when describing structures on the head, since the word cranial cannot be used, and indicates that something is closer to the nose, or further forward.

Body fluid compartments

4. C   The anion found in common salt is chloride

Common salt is more technically called sodium chloride, and when this is dissolved in water it separates into two ions – the sodium and chloride ions. Each carries a charge; sodium positive (Na^+) and chloride negative (Cl^-). The terms anion and cation relate to the type of charge; anions are negatively charged, and cations positive.

5. B   66% of the total body water is found within cells

Fluid makes up 60-80% of an animal's bodyweight, and of this fluid two-thirds or 66% is found within cells.

Some texts express this in a different way, relating the fluids in each compartment to the animal's bodyweight:

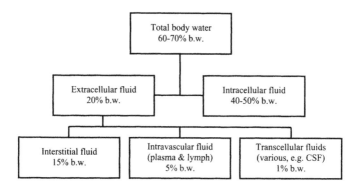

Note that lymph should be included in the intravascular section, since this is in direct communication with the bloodstream.

This method is useful when it comes to considering fluid therapy, so that it can be determined how much of a fluid deficit has been lost from the circulation.

6. C   The heart is not involved in the regulation of pH within the body

pH is a measure of the level of acidity of a substance. Anything described as acidic contains large numbers of free hydrogen ions. It is very important that the pH of blood and tissues is maintained by the body so that enzymes are able to function optimally. Blood normally has a pH of 7.4, and there are several ways in which this is kept constant:

- The lungs are used to control the levels of carbon dioxide in the body. Carbon dioxide dissolves in water to give carbonic acid, which therefore affects the pH of the fluid.
- The kidneys control not just fluid levels within the body but also the acid-base balance. Hydrogen ions can be excreted by the distal convoluted tubule of the kidneys to raise pH.
- Plasma contains proteins which are able to loosely combine with hydrogen ions, and therefore reduce their effect on plasma pH. These proteins are often referred to as buffers, since if acid levels fall, then the protein-hydrogen ion pairing will separate and ensure that free hydrogen ion levels stay as constant as possible.

7. B   The solution with pH 5.5 is the most acidic

As mentioned in question 6, the pH scale is used to describe the concentration of hydrogen ions in a solution. The scale runs from 0 to 14. An acidic solution with high hydrogen ion concentration has a pH less than 7, whereas an alkaline (also referred to as basic) solution has a pH of over 7. Solutions such as pure water, with pH 7, are neutral.

8. D   An average animal will lose 20 ml/kg/24 hours through respiration

Respiration results in quite considerable fluid losses over time, and these should always be taken into account when estimating an animal's fluid requirements. Other normal routes of fluid loss include urine and faeces. Note that sweat is considered to be negligible.

9. B   A solution which exerts a higher osmotic pressure than plasma is hypertonic

Solutions with the same osmotic pressure are isotonic, and those with lower osmotic pressure are hypotonic.

Hyperbaric refers to a different type of pressure: the force exerted due to the pressure of a fluid or gas within a container. The term is most usually used in relation to hyperbaric chambers which contain oxygen at high pressure. It is not something that applies particularly to veterinary medicine.

10. D   The main anion within intracellular fluid is phosphate

Phosphate is the most important anion in cells, since it is needed to enable the cell to produce adenosine triphosphate (ATP). The main intracellular cation is potassium. Outside the cell the composition is quite different – there are very few proteins, the main cation is the sodium ion, and the main anion, chloride.

The difference in composition is maintained by proteins in the wall of cells, such as the sodium-potassium pump. This maintains the differing composition by pumping sodium ions out of cells, and in exchange bringing in potassium ions.

Cell structure

11. C   Adenosine triphosphate (ATP) is formed within cells by mitochondria

All organelles in the cell have specific functions. Mitochondria produce the energy needed for the cell, and they do this by creating high energy molecules, namely ATP molecules. When the cell needs energy it breaks down these molecules to produce ADP (adenosine diphosphate) and energy, which is then used by the cell.

Ribosomes are responsible for protein synthesis within the cell.

Vacuoles are membrane-bound cavities found within the cytoplasm of cells.

Centrioles are structures which act as the centres for the mitotic spindle which is formed during cell division.

12. A   The four stages of mitosis in order are: prophase, metaphase, anaphase, telophase

Prophase is the first stage, and this is when the nuclear membrane breaks down, and the chromosomes condense, becoming visible under the microscope. Metaphase follows, during which the chromosomes start to arrange themselves along the mitotic spindle ready to separate. During anaphase the chromosomes are pulled to the opposite ends of the cell, and in telophase the final separation of the two cells occurs, and the nuclear membrane reforms in each.

13. A   Phagocytosis describes the way in which some cells are able to engulf solid particles

Not all cells are able to do this, but cells such as monocytes and neutrophils (two of the white blood cells) use this to the animal's advantage by removing foreign particles, cell debris and bacteria.

Pinocytosis describes the way in which cells can take up liquids.

Exocytosis is the expulsion of small particles by the cell.

14. C   **The organelle responsible for transporting materials around the cell is the endoplasmic reticulum**

The endoplasmic reticulum consists of a system of membranes, and is used to transport a variety of substances around the cell.

The golgi apparatus produces some of the secretions made by cells, and is also involved in the production of lysosomes.

Lysosomes are vacuoles (membrane-bound pockets) that contain digestive enzymes. When material is phagocytosed it is brought into the lysosome and the enzymes then break it down.

15. B   **Interphase is the stage in the cell cycle during which the cell rests between cell divisions**

The four main stages of mitosis are those described in question 12; prophase, metaphase, anaphase and telophase. Once a cell completes telophase, and the nuclear membrane has reformed, the cell enters interphase – the stage between successive cell divisions.

Basic tissue types

16. A   Tendon is an example of a dense connective tissue

Connective tissues are divided into a number of different types depending on the substance or matrix found between the cells and fibres that make up the tissue.

Some connective tissues are solid, such as bone, whereas others are less rigid, such as cartilage or the dense connective tissues.

Dense connective tissues vary in function, but tendons and ligaments, which contain large numbers of fibres come into this category, and their role is to attach muscles to bone, or bone to bone. The fibres are all lined up in the direction of pull, in order to give the tissues additional strength.

Adipose tissue is less organised, and is described as a loose connective tissue. It contains large numbers of fat cells and has several functions. It acts as an energy store, it provides protection for delicate organs and it insulates the animal's body.

17. D   Areolar tissue is found beneath skin and is used as a packing material in the body

Areolar tissue is loose connective tissue, and is found in many sites in the body as a space filler. It is easily cut through, and is most commonly seen during operations as the tissue immediately underneath the skin. Surgeons usually break down this tissue by blunt dissection when separating skin from the underlying muscles.

Adipose tissue is also a loose connective tissue, and it is this tissue that contains large numbers of fat cells. It serves to provide not only an energy store, but also insulation for the animal and protection of certain organs.

18. A   Blood vessels are lined by simple squamous epithelium

This is the thinnest type of epithelium, and is found wherever diffusion occurs. Nutrients have to be able to diffuse through capillary walls to reach the body's cells. Hence they are made of this type of epithelium. Larger blood vessels are still lined with squamous epithelium, but there are additional layers of tissue outside the lining.

Stratified squamous epithelium is found where protection is required – such as the skin. Stratified epithelia are made of a number of layers of cells.

Transitional epithelium is also a type of stratified epithelium, but this has the additional property of being able to stretch. This is found in the bladder and urethra.

Cuboidal epithelium is most usually found lining glands and ducts.

19. B   The type of cartilage found in the intervertebral discs is fibrocartilage

The different types of cartilage have differing functions and are therefore found in different locations within the body. Hyaline cartilage is found covering the articular surface of bones, and also forms the rings of the trachea. Elastic cartilage is more flexible, and the sites where it is found, such as the pinna of the ear and the laryngeal cartilages, reflect this.

The body cavities

20. C **The pleura lining the inside of the ribcage is called the costal pleura**

Pleura is the name given to the serous membranes lining the thoracic cavity. There are two pleural sacs, and the membranes are given different names depending which structures the membrane is closest to.

Parietal pleura is a general term used to describe the membrane lining the boundaries of the thorax. Visceral pleura is also a general term, and refers to the membrane covering organs.

Diaphragmatic pleura covers the diaphragm, and is part of the parietal pleura, as is the costal pleura.

Pulmonary pleura covers the lungs and so this is therefore part of the visceral portion of the membrane.

21. C **The kidney is retroperitoneal**

Retroperitoneal literally means behind the peritoneum. The kidney sits close to the abdominal wall, and is therefore only covered in peritoneum on one side.

22. A **The azygous vein is found in the mediastinum**

The mediastinum is the space formed between the right and left pleural cavities, which contains the major blood vessels in the thorax and the oesophagus.

The prostate and spleen are both found in the abdomen, and are therefore covered in peritoneum. The thyroid gland is found in the neck, and therefore not coated with serous membrane.

23. C **Mesentery is best described as the peritoneal fold which lies between the abdominal wall and the intestine**

The main body cavities are lined with serous membranes. In the thorax there are two pleural membranes, and in the abdomen one peritoneal membrane. Terms are used to describe specific areas of these membranes.

The space between the right and left pleural membranes is the mediastinum.

The peritoneal fold between the abdominal wall and the stomach is the omentum.

The fold of peritoneum between the uterus and the body wall is the broad ligament.

The skeletal system

24. C   **Mast cells are not found associated with the skeletal system**

The skeleton contains a number of different cell types.

Osteoblasts are the cells that actively lay down new bone matrix; osteoclasts are the cells that break down the matrix. Both types are active throughout an animal's life, so bones are subject to constant remodelling. Chondrocytes are needed to produce both the initial cartilage model for bones that form by endochondral ossification, and to produce the cartilage that covers the articular surfaces of bones.

Mast cells contain histamine and are found in loose connective tissue. They release histamine when the tissue is damaged, and this stimulates an inflammatory response.

25. D   **The bones that form by intramembranous ossification are flat bones**

Sesamoid bones form within the tendons of muscles.
The splanchnic skeleton forms within soft tissue structures.
Long bones form by enchondral ossification.

26. C   **The shaft of the bone is known as the diaphysis**

Several different terms are used to describe specific regions of the long bones. The end of the bone is the epiphysis, the growth plate region of a bone is the physis, and the area adjacent to this, where new bone is being laid down, is the metaphysis. Finally, the cavity within the bone is the medullary cavity.

27. A   **The parietal bone is an example of a flat bone**

The atlas can be described as an irregular bone, due to its unusual shape. The tibia is a long bone, and the patella is a sesamoid bone, since this forms within the tendon of insertion of the quadriceps femoris muscle.

28. B   The pubis does not form part of the axial skeleton

The axial skeleton consists of all the bones that make up the linear framework of the body, whereas the appendicular skeleton consists of the limbs. Thus the axial skeleton includes the skull, vertebrae, ribs and sternum, and the appendicular skeleton includes all the other bones of the skeleton.

29. D   The os penis is part of the splanchnic skeleton

The splanchnic skeleton consists of bones which form in soft tissues and are unconnected with the rest of the skeleton. The os penis is the only bone of significance in this category in small animals.

The fabellae are similar to the patella, in that they too are sesamoid bones. There are two in each leg, and they form in the tendons of origin of the gastrocnemius muscle.

The frontal bone is part of the axial skeleton and the femur is part of the appendicular skeleton.

30. C   The sphenoid bone forms the floor of the cranium

The sphenoid bone (also called the sphenoidal bone) is found in the midline on the underside of the skull. Some people subdivide this into two bones, one in front of the other, and call these the presphenoid and the basisphenoid, so you may find it referred to like this in some texts.

The frontal and temporal bones are both paired (i.e. there is one on each side of the head). The frontal bones form the 'forehead' region of the skull and contain the frontal sinuses. The temporal bones are totally irregular in shape. They form part of the lateral wall of the cranium, house the middle ear within the tympanic bulla, and have a prominence that extends rostrally to meet the zygomatic bone to form the zygomatic arch.

The occipital bone, like the sphenoid bone, is unpaired. This forms the caudal boundary of the cranium, and in its centre is the large foramen magnum through which the spinal cord passes.

31. B   The maxilla contains a sinus

A sinus is an air-filled chamber within the bone, and there are two bones in the skull which contain these: the maxilla and the frontal bones. Together the maxillary and frontal sinuses are referred to as the paranasal sinuses.

32. D   The statement 'The largest vertebrae in the spine are the 7 lumbar vertebrae' is correct

All the other statements are untrue:

There are 7 cervical vertebrae not 5.

The 3 sacral vertebrae are fused in both cats and dogs.

The coccygeal vertebrae can also be called caudal vertebrae.

33. A   The term used to describe a long thin skull is doliocephalic

A standard-shaped skull, such as that of a Labrador, is described either as mesocephalic or mesaticephalic, and a short-nosed animal, such as a Pug or Persian cat, is brachycephalic.

34. B   Fovea are found on the thoracic vertebrae

The fovea on the 13 thoracic vertebrae are flattened areas on the transverse processes where the tubercles of the ribs articulate.

This is one of two joints formed between each vertebrae and rib – the other is on the body of the vertebra where head of the rib has its articulation. Both joints are synovial joints.

35. D   The fabellae are located adjacent to the stifle

The fabellae are two small sesamoid bones which form in the tendons of origin of the gastrocnemius muscle. The origin of each head of the muscle is on the caudal aspect of the distal femur, so the two bones are found just caudal to the stifle joint. They may show quite clearly on radiographs of the stifle, and should not be confused with fracture fragments.

Answers

36. A   The large bone that forms the point of the hock is the calcaneus

This bone has several names – calcaneus is one, but it is also referred to as the os calcis or the fibular tarsal bone, and students should be aware of this, since anatomy texts often vary which term is used.

The talus is the other bone in the proximal row of tarsal bones. This also has another name – the tibial tarsal bone.

In the forelimb there is an accessory carpal bone, but there is no accessory tarsal bone in the hind leg.

37. A   Flexion describes movement of a joint in which the angle between the two bones is reduced

The opposite movement is extension, i.e. the joint is straightened.

If a whole limb is swung forward in a cranial direction, then the movement is described as protraction. Movement in a caudal direction is retraction.

Abduction and adduction describe movement of a limb away from and towards the midline.

38. C   The greater trochanter is found on the femur

This is the prominent bulge on the lateral aspect of the proximal femur, and is an important site of muscle attachment. It can also be palpated quite readily, and is a useful bony landmark when radiographing the pelvis and hindlimb.

The equivalent in the foreleg is the greater tubercle, found on the humerus.

The tibia has a tuberosity on its cranial surface where quadriceps femoris attaches.

The radius comes to a point at its distal end which is called the styloid process.

39. A   The type of joint that allows the most movement is a diarthrosis

Diarthroses are the moving joints of the body and are also called synovial joints, since these are lubricated by synovial fluid within a joint capsule.

Amphiarthroses, such as intervertebral discs, and symphyses, such as the pubic and mandibular symphyses allow only a small amount of movement or 'give'.

Synarthroses are fused joints, and the best examples of these are the sutures found between the flat bones of the skull.

The muscular system

40. B   **Skeletal muscle can also be described as striated muscle**

If skeletal muscle is examined microscopically, then bands or striations can be seen across the muscle cells where the actin and myosin fibrils overlap.

Smooth muscle (also called visceral muscle) also has the protein fibres, but they are not arranged regularly, and so the areas of overlap are not visible under the light microscope.

Cardiac muscle does not have any alternative names.

41. D   **A motor unit is defined as a group of muscle cells supplied by one nerve fibre**

Motor units are variable in size depending on the level of control needed for a particular muscle. Thus the motor units in a powerful muscle such as the limb muscles are large, consisting of several hundred muscle cells. However, in muscles needing very fine control, such as the small muscles controlling eye movement, the motor units are much smaller, consisting of only a few muscle cells in each.

42. D   **The prime protractor of the forelimb is brachiocephalicus**

Protraction describes the movement of the whole limb in a forward direction. This occurs in walking when the animal swings its leg forwards before placing it on the ground. Trapezius also plays a role in this movement, but is far less powerful than brachiocephalicus.

The other muscles have actions as follows:

Biceps femoris is found on the hindlimb, and has several actions including hip extension, stifle flexion and hock extension.

Brachialis and biceps brachii are both found on the front leg, and both cause elbow flexion. Of the two, biceps brachii is the stronger and more important.

43. A   Trapezius is an extrinsic muscle of the forelimb

A muscle is described as extrinsic if its origin and insertion cross from one part of the body to another, for example from the trunk to the limb, as in this example. Trapezius has its origin on the spinous processes of thoracic vertebrae, and its insertion on the scapula.

The other muscles all link one forelimb bone to another, and are therefore described as intrinsic muscles of the forelimb.

44. A   The muscle never involved in respiration is latissimus dorsi

Although this muscle lies across the thorax, its function is to move the forelimb, and it is never involved in respiratory function.

The abdominal muscles such as external abdominal oblique and transversus abdominis occasionally assist in laboured breathing, and both internal and external intercostals are used in normal respiration.

45. D   Extension of the elbow is caused by triceps brachii

Brachialis and biceps brachii both affect the elbow joint, but are elbow flexors, and supraspinatus is a shoulder extensor.

46. A   Latissimus dorsi has its origin on the spinous processes of the thoracic vertebrae

Latissimus dorsi is the main forelimb retractor. Pectineus is found in the hindlimb and is an adductor. Infraspinatus links the scapula to the humerus, and semimembranosus, along with biceps femoris and semitendinosus, makes up the hamstrings on the caudal aspect of the thigh.

47. B   The tendon of anterior tibial does not form part of the Achilles tendon

The Achilles tendon, which leads to the point of the hock, is made up of the tendons of four muscles – biceps femoris, semitendinosus, gastrocnemius and superficial digital flexor.

48. B Within a muscle cell there are filaments which slide over each other when a muscle cell contracts

These filaments are made of proteins called actin and myosin. There needs to be a supply of free calcium ions within the cell for muscle contraction to occur, and available energy in the form of ATP.

A sarcomere is the name given to the unit of muscle contraction – in each sarcomere there is a set of actin and myosin filaments, and when the muscle contracts the two ends of each unit are pulled closer together.

49. D Rectus abdominis has its insertion on the pelvis via the prepubic tendon

The other muscles run in different directions – the obliques both have fibres running on opposite diagonals and transversus abdominis runs across the abdomen. These three muscles insert via the linea alba, an aponeurosis (tendon sheet) found in the midline of the animal.

50. B Gastrocnemius is a stifle flexor and hock extensor

Gastrocnemius lies on the caudal aspect of the limb and is often referred to as the calf muscle. It has its origin on the distal femur, and then inserts via the Achilles tendon on the calcaneus (os calcis). When it contracts, it affects both the stifle and hock joint, causing the movements listed above.

The nervous system

51. C   'A neuron has only one axon' is the true statement

Neurons or nerve cells have slightly different structures depending on where they are found in the nervous system, and what their role is. There are neurons, such as intercalated neurons, which do not have dendrites, so A cannot be true. The neurons that do have dendrites use these cytoplasmic outgrowths to carry impulses towards the cell body, not as stated in B away from the cell. Some neurons, particularly those found in lower species, do not have myelin covering the surfaces of the axons. These conduct impulses more slowly than myelinated cells, but nevertheless are still functional.

52. C   A synapse is found between two neurons

A synapse is the connection formed between two neurons. The central canal simply contains cerebro-spinal fluid, and the dorsal root ganglion contains only the cell bodies of sensory neurons. There are no neuron connections at this site.

53. A   The parasympathetic nervous system stimulates salivation

The parasympathetic nervous system deals with many routine body functions, including gut movement, urination, defaecation, lacrimation and salivation, and slows the heart rate.

The sympathetic nervous system prepares the body for action, the so-called 'flight or fight' response, and the best way to envisage the effects of the sympathetic nervous system is to think of a scared cat! The fur stands on end, the pupils are widely dilated, the heart rate is very fast, and blood has been directed away from skin and intestines through vasoconstriction, and shunted towards the muscles and brain ready for action.

54. A   The CNS develops from the ectodermal layer of the inner cell mass

The mesoderm forms the musculo-skeletal system and internal organs. The endoderm gives rise to the lining of the digestive tract and other visceral organs.

The trophoblast develops into the extra-embryonic membranes, which include the tissues that will form part of the placenta, and the membranes that protect the embryo during its development.

55. A   The part of the brain responsible for conscious thought is the cerebrum

The cerebrum consists of the two cerebral hemispheres and forms the bulk of the forebrain. This is where all the senses are perceived, and where conscious thought takes place.

The hypothalamus is a small area of the forebrain which has several roles. One of these is to provide communication between the nervous system and the endocrine system, by stimulating the pituitary gland to secrete hormones in response to detected changes in the body. It is also is very important in regulating homeostatic mechanisms and helps to control the autonomic nervous system.

The cerebellum and medulla oblongata are both part of the hindbrain. The main function of the cerebellum is to coordinate balance and movement, whereas the medulla is concerned with basic reflex activities such as respiration and maintenance of blood pressure.

56. B   The cerebral aqueduct is found within the midbrain

In the centre of the central nervous system are a series of channels and chambers within which is cerebro-spinal fluid (CSF), which helps to protect the brain and spinal cord from trauma.

In the forebrain there are three chambers, the two lateral ventricles and the third ventricle. The fluid continues through the midbrain in the cerebral aqueduct to the hindbrain where the fourth ventricle is found. A small channel – the central canal – continues caudally into the spinal cord.

57. D   Nociceptors are found in skin

These are pain receptors, and are found not only in skin, but throughout the tissues of the body.

Proprioceptors provide information about the position and attitude of the body and include a number of different types of receptor. Examples include joint receptors and the vestibular apparatus.

Chemoreceptors are used to detect the concentration of specific chemicals within the body, and baroreceptors respond to blood pressure.

58. A   The cranial nerve that carries parasympathetic neurons to the head is cranial nerve III, the oculomotor nerve

Parasympathetic neurons have a cranio-sacral outflow, which means that they only emerge from the central nervous system with cranial and sacral nerves. However, not all cranial nerves carry parasympathetic neurons – cranial nerve III takes parasympathetic neurons to the eye, where their effects include pupil dilation and lacrimation. Cranial nerves IV and VIII do not carry any parasympathetic neurons, and although the vagus is very important, carrying parasympathetic neurons to the thorax and abdomen, it does not actually supply any tissues around the head with this type of nerve supply.

59. C   The vestibulo-cochlear nerve conveys the sense of hearing

Only two of the nerves listed actually exist. There is neither an auditory nerve nor a cerebellar nerve.

The vagus nerve does exist, but this is involved in supplying tissues of the head and neck with somatic motor neurons, and parasympathetic neurons to the thorax and abdomen.

60. C   Sympathetic neurons leave the central nervous system via thoracic and lumbar nerves

There are no sympathetic neurons in the cranial nerves, cervical nerves or sacral nerves. However, both the cranial and caudal ends of the animal do receive sympathetic supply via the sympathetic chain.

61. C   The term plexus describes a network

The word plexus appears in a number of different contexts, but in each case it refers to a network of structures. In the nervous system, the brachial plexus describes a network of nerves found in the axilla region. A blood vessel network can also be termed a plexus, such as the choroid plexuses found in the ventricles of the brain which produce the cerebro-spinal fluid.

62. B   The neurotransmitter used by the parasympathetic nervous system is acetyl choline

There are a number of chemicals used as neurotransmitters within the nervous system. Dopamine is an important transmitter found within many nerve cells of the brain. Acetyl choline is found both in parasympathetic neurons and somatic neurons, and noradrenaline is found within the end terminals of sympathetic nerve cells.

63. A   An afferent somatic neuron is a sensory neuron

The terms afferent and efferent can be used to describe the direction of nerve impulses with respect to the central nervous system. Afferent literally means carrying towards, so a neuron carrying impulses towards the CNS is bringing in sensory information. Motor neurons can therefore be called efferent neurons since they carry impulses away from the CNS.

Intercalated neurons are only found in the CNS, and act as linking neurons between the motor and sensory parts of the nervous system.

64. B   Gustation is another word for taste

Smell can also be referred to as olfaction. Swallowing is also called deglutition, and there is no other word for digestion.

65. A   The limbus is the junction between the sclera and the cornea

The other terms that you should be aware of are:

- The area where the lacrimal gland opens is called the fornix
- The point at which upper and lower eyelids meet is the canthus.

66. B   Animals focus light onto the retina by altering the pull on the lens via the suspensory ligament and ciliary body

In order to focus light onto the retina, the light must undergo refraction or bending. The amount of bending needed varies with how far away the object being looked at is. Near objects require more refraction to bring them into focus than far ones. Light is refracted in the eye at the front and back surfaces of the cornea and at the front and back of the lens. Altering the pull on the lens alters its shape slightly, and this in turn affects how much refraction takes place. The ability to focus images is called accommodation.

The size of the pupil is also important for vision, but this does not affect the animal's ability to focus, just to control how much light actually gets through to the retina. The size varies with ambient light levels.

Neither the curvature of the cornea nor the density of the aqueous humour are altered in a normal eye.

67. D   The pupil is not part of the uvea

The uvea consists of three structures found within the eye: the choroid, the iris and the ciliary body. All are pigmented and vascular.

The choroid is the pigmented layer found behind the retina. Most of this layer contains dark pigment, but there is a region close to the optic disc where the pigment is reflective. This is the tapetum or tapetum lucidum.

The iris is the obviously coloured part of the eye, and smooth muscles within this contract or relax to alter the size of the hole in the middle – the pupil.

The ciliary body also contains smooth muscle which contracts or relaxes to alter the pull on the lens and change focal distance.

68. C **Salivation at the sight of the fridge being opened is a conditional reflex**

Conditional reflexes are learned reflexes, that take place when associations are made between an action that would not normally elicit a response with one that would. Salivation is usually associated with the sight, smell or taste of food. However, animals quickly learn if the fridge contains their food, and will therefore respond to the door being opened even though they have not yet even seen or smelt the food.

The other reflexes described are all unconditional reflexes, and would be reproducible in a wide range of animals and species. In these, the stimulus and response are directly linked.

The names for each reflex in order are A the patella reflex, B the panninculus reflex and D the withdrawal or pedal reflex.

69. A **The function of the ossicles is to transmit sound waves across the middle ear cavity**

The three ossicles (malleus, incus and stapes) form a bridge between the tympanic membrane and the oval window. Sound waves impinge on the tympanic membrane which causes malleus to vibrate. This in turn pushes incus, which causes stapes to move. The stapes bone sits against the oval window, a membrane separating the middle and inner ear cavities, and causes this to vibrate. Therefore, movements of the tympanic membrane are transferred across the middle ear cavity to the inner ear.

The semicircular canals within the inner ear are responsible for the detection of head movement, and the otolith organs detect head position.

The eustachian tube provides the link between the middle ear and the naso-pharynx. This is usually kept closed but opens during swallowing or yawning to allow the air pressure within the middle ear to become the same as that in the nasal chambers.

70. B   The vestibular apparatus is made up of the otolith organs and the semicircular canals

The vestibular apparatus is housed within the inner ear and is concerned with proprioception. There are two parts – the semicircular canals which detect head movement, and the otolith organs (the utricle and saccule) which give information about head position. Impulses are relayed to the brain via the vestibulo-cochlear nerve.

The external ear canal and pinna form the outer ear, and are responsible for directing sound waves towards the tympanic membrane.

The ossicles transmit the sound waves across the middle ear and the organ of Corti within the inner ear detects sound waves. This too uses the vestibulo-cochlear nerve to send the information to the brain.

Finally, the eustachian tube acts as described in the answer to question 69, to equalise air pressure in the middle ear.

The endocrine system

71. A The function of chorionic gonadotrophin is to maintain the corpus luteum

It is important that the corpus luteum stays active during the pregnancy, since it secretes progesterone needed to ensure that the uterine wall is prepared ready for implantation of the embryo. The progesterone also provides feedback to the pituitary, preventing the release of follicle stimulating hormone and luteinising hormone, and stopping the animal from entering her next oestrous cycle.

72. B Adrenocorticotrophic hormone (ACTH) is secreted by the anterior pituitary

ACTH is produced during times of stress, and stimulates the adrenal cortex to produce glucocorticoids such as cortisol.

Aldosterone is a second type of hormone secreted by the adrenal cortex, and is involved with sodium balance in the body.

Oestrogen is secreted by the Graaffian follicles formed within the ovary. This is responsible for the physical and behavioural signs seen in oestrus.

Parathyroid hormone (PTH) is secreted by the parathyroid glands. PTH is involved in regulation of blood calcium levels.

73. A Mammary glands do not contain endocrine tissue

The other organs all do. The kidney secretes two hormones – erythropoietin required for red blood cell maturation, and renin which stimulates the conversion of angiotensinogen into angiotensin. The small intestine produces secretin, needed to stimulate the pancreas and gall bladder to release their digestive secretions, and the pancreas secretes several hormones including insulin and glucagon.

74. D   Addison's disease is caused by lack of mineralocorticoids

Addison's disease, or hypoadrenocorticism, results from the lack of mineralocorticoids produced by the adrenal cortex. The main hormone involved is aldosterone, and this normally causes sodium retention when it is released. Animals without aldosterone cannot regulate sodium levels fully. The sodium-potassium ratio within the extracellular fluids is altered and this leads to marked abnormalities in fluid balance. This condition is serious, and animals should be treated as soon as possible.

Lack of ADH causes diabetes insipidus, and the animal is unable to concentrate its urine.

The opposite to Addison's disease is hyperadrenocorticism, or Cushing's disease, where the signs seen are due to over-production of the corticosteroids.

Finally, lack of growth hormone leads to dwarfism.

75. D   The hormone that regulates metabolic rate is thyroxine

Thyroxine (thyroid hormone) is produced by the thyroid gland and determines the metabolic rate of an individual. It is also essential for normal growth.

76. C   Oxytocin is produced by the posterior pituitary

Oxytocin is an ecbolic, stimulating uterine contractions. It is also required for initial milk let-down after the young have been born.

77. A   The function of interstitial cell stimulating hormone is to stimulate the release of testosterone from the cells of Leydig

The cells of Leydig in the testes are also called the interstitial cells, and they secrete testosterone needed for spermatogenesis and the development of secondary sexual characteristics in the male.

The pancreas does secrete somatostatin, which helps to smooth out swings in blood glucose levels, but this is not under hormonal control.

Follicle stimulating hormone (FSH) is required for follicle development, and aldosterone is the hormone responsible for stimulating the kidney to reabsorb sodium.

78. C   The hormone normally released when blood calcium levels rise above normal is thyrocalcitonin

If calcium levels rise above normal, the body needs to deposit some of the calcium in bone. Thyrocalcitonin (or calcitonin) stimulates osteoblast activity and encourages bone matrix deposition.

Parathyroid hormone does the opposite. It is released when calcium levels fall, and it stimulates osteoclast activity. These cells break down bone matrix to release calcium into the bloodstream.

Thyrocalcitonin is produced by the thyroid glands, but the other hormone secreted by the thyroids, thyroid hormone or thyroxine, has no real effect on calcium levels. It is, however, very important for regulation of metabolic rate.

Glucagon is a hormone released by the pancreas, and it acts to cause glycogen breakdown in the liver, and to reduce glucose uptake by cells. This therefore prevents glucose levels in the bloodstream from falling too low.

The blood vascular system

79. B **The removal of excess interstitial fluid from the spaces between cells to prevent the development of oedema is not a function of the bloodstream**

When blood passes through the capillaries, some fluid is squeezed out into the interstitial spaces. Most returns to the bloodstream due to the osmotic effect of plasma proteins, but some tends to remain within the interstitial spaces. This fluid is collected within the lymph capillaries, and carried to larger lymph vessels before it is eventually returned to the circulation close to the heart.

The bloodstream carries out all the other functions listed in the question.

80. C **The pH of blood is 7.4**

This is important since it is the pH that enables the body's enzymes to work optimally. If it changes it can have serious effects.

81. A **The smallest blood cell found in the circulation is the erythrocyte**

Erythrocytes are smaller than any of the white blood cells. The only smaller cellular components in blood are thrombocytes.

The lymphocyte is the smallest of the white cells; the granulocytes are slightly larger, and the monocytes are the largest of the leucocytes.

82. B **The hormone erythropoietin is produced by the kidney**

Erythropoietin is needed for maturation of red blood cells as they develop within the bone marrow.

83. A **The white blood cell with granules in its cytoplasm containing histamine is the basophil**

The granulocytes, neutrophils, eosinophils and basophils,

all contain granules containing different chemicals with different staining characteristics. Histamine is alkaline and therefore takes up the methylene blue from Romanowsky stains. Eosinophils have acidic granules which take up the red dye, eosin, and neutrophils have neutral granules which do not take up either stain.

84. A   The white blood cells responsible for the production of antibodies are B-lymphocytes

All the white cells have protective roles within the bloodstream, but these vary from cell to cell. Lymphocytes are divided into two types with B-lymphocytes being responsible for the humoral immune response (production of antibodies), and T-lymphocytes responsible for the cell-mediated immune response.

Neutrophils and monocytes are both phagocytes; neutrophils remove bacteria particularly, whereas monocytes remove cell debris and other foreign material.

85. D   The cells in which Howell-Jolly bodies are seen are reticulocytes

Reticulocytes are immature red blood cells that have been pushed out into the circulation slightly before they are ready. They are normally seen in anaemia, since an immature red blood cell can still carry some oxygen, and support the animal. The Howell-Jolly bodies are the remnants of organelles including the nucleus that are normally removed from the erythrocytes as they mature.

86. C   The epicardium is a serous membrane

The heart is made up of several different tissues. On the inside is the endocardium, an epithelial layer. Next is the myocardium, the heart muscle, and covering this is the epicardium, which is strictly part of the pericardium. The epicardium secretes serous fluid into a small cavity between this layer and the rest of the pericardium. This cavity is the pericardial cavity and the fluid is pericardial fluid.

The chordae tendineae are fibres which attach to the valve leaflets and prevent them being turned inside out.

87. B   The bicuspid valve is also called the mitral valve

Several of the valves have more than one name, and it is important that you are aware of this, since it can be confusing when trying to decipher a case history.

88. A   It is true that deoxygenated blood returns to the heart from the body via the vena cava

Oxygenated blood returns to the heart from the lungs via the pulmonary vein, not the pulmonary artery.

Deoxygenated blood flows through the right side of the heart not the left.

Deoxygenated blood leaves the heart for the lungs via the pulmonary artery, not the aorta.

89. C   Purkinje fibres are specialised conducting cells which spread the wave of contraction through the walls of the ventricles

When the heart contracts, waves of contractions originate from the sino-atrial node in the right atrium of the heart, and progress through the heart. Heart muscle cells are unusual since there are electrical connections or intercalated discs between adjacent cells, and when one starts to contract it triggers the next cell in line to contract. However, in order to get synchronous contraction of the ventricles, there have to be faster conduction routes through the walls of the ventricles. These include the Purkinje fibres.

There are fibres connecting the valve leaflets, but these are totally unrelated to the Purkinje fibres and are called the chordae tendineae. These have no electrical activity.

90. D   The first heart sound, lubb, is the sound of the atrio-ventricular valves closing

There are two heart sounds – lubb and dub. The first sound occurs as the ventricles start to contract (systole) and blood starts to try to flow back into the atria. This forces the valves to close.

The second sound occurs when the ventricles relax

(diastole), and the blood tends to try to flow back into the ventricles from the arteries which forces the aortic and pulmonic valves shut. These valves are sometimes referred to as the semilunar valves.

Thus the two atrio-ventricular valves (tricupsid and mitral) should always close together, and the same is true for the two semilunar valves, but the tricupsid valve could never close at the same time as the aortic valve.

91. B   The artery that carries blood to the stomach, spleen and liver is the coeliac artery

There are two coronary arteries and these supply the heart muscle.

The cranial mesenteric artery is found in the cranial part of the abdomen, and this supplies the small intestine.

The subclavian arteries branch off the aorta, and curl around the front of the shoulder joint under the clavicle (if present) on each side. The arteries then continue down each foreleg as the axillary arteries and the brachial arteries.

92. D   All the statements are true

Lymph vessels and veins are quite similar in structure and function. Both carry fluid back towards the heart, and since this fluid has already been to tissues, it is deoxygenated. The walls of the vessels are fairly thin, and fluid movement depends on a number of factors including muscle activity. Since they are low pressure vessels, backflow would be possible except that both have valves incorporated to prevent this.

93. B   The hepatic portal vein connects the capillary network of the intestines and the liver

Portal veins are unusual in that they connect two capillary beds. Normally veins are found between capillaries and larger veins, but the hepatic portal vein ensures that nutrients absorbed by the small intestine into the bloodstream are able to go directly to the liver for processing.

94. D   It is not normal to be able to palpate the retropharyngeal lymph nodes

As the name suggests, these lymph nodes are found caudal to the pharynx, and are only palpable when they have reached a very large size, and are starting to put pressure on the oesophagus and larynx.

95. B   The spleen contains both lymphoid and myeloid tissue

There are two types of haemopoietic tissue in the body – lymphoid and myeloid tissue. Myeloid tissue produces red blood cells and most of the white blood cells. Lymphoid tissue produces lymphocytes and is also responsible for filtering lymph fluid before it is returned to the blood circulation.

Bone marrow only contains myeloid tissue, and the thymus and lymph nodes contain just lymphoid tissue.

The respiratory system

96. A **The sequence in which air passes through the structures on its way to the lungs is nares, pharynx, larynx, trachea, bronchi, bronchioles**

97. C **Sounds are produced in the larynx**

Vocalisation occurs when air passes the vocal folds which project into the larynx. They consist of a pair of vocal ligaments which are covered in mucous membranes. The vibration of the folds causes the production of sounds, and the 'voice' of every animal and person is a unique mix of vibrations.

98. B **The opening into the larynx is the glottis**

The larynx is made up of a number of cartilages linked by muscle and covered in mucous membrane. It leads to the trachea, and it is therefore imperative that substances other than air do not enter the larynx. The epiglottis is a flap of cartilage that is pushed against the glottis to seal it closed during swallowing, and this prevents aspiration of food and liquid.

99. D **The true statement is that the right lung has an accessory lobe**

The two lungs are not exactly equal. The right lung has 4 lobes – cranial, middle, caudal and accessory lobes, whereas the left has only 3 (no accessory lobe).

Alternate names for the lobes are occasionally used. The cranial lobe is the apical lobe, the middle lobe is the cardiac lobeand the caudal lobe is the diaphragmatic lobe.

100. C **The term 'dead space' refers to the parts of the respiratory tract where gaseous exchange does not occur**

Gaseous exchange only takes place in the alveoli, but to get there the air has to be moved through the rest of the respiratory tract. Air in this part of the tract is not usable, and is therefore 'dead'.

The space between the lungs and the thoracic wall is the pleural cavity. This should normally be very small since it is bounded by the parietal and pulmonary pleura, and there is a slight negative pressure within it which encourages the lungs to remain inflated.

101. A   The breathing centres that control the basic breathing cycle are located in the hindbrain

There are a couple of breathing centres found in the hindbrain and these allow for regular respiration without conscious thought being required. However, higher centres in the brain can also influence the breathing pattern, since it is possible to breath-hold deliberately, and also other factors such as stress and pain can alter the way in which animals and people breathe.

102. C   It is untrue that oxygen is the most important factor in determining respiratory rate

There are many factors that control respiratory rate, including emotional as well as physical factors. Carbon dioxide levels are one of the most important influences, since a build up of carbon dioxide in the blood lowers pH, and leads to acidosis which can be fatal. The other statements are all true.

103. D   The term that describes the volume of air that is exhaled during forceful expiration after maximum inspiration is vital capacity

Tidal volume refers to the amount of air moved in and out of the lungs during normal breathing. Not all air is exhaled during breathing, and the baseline volume left in the lungs after relaxed expiration is the functional residual capacity.

Even if an animal or person exhales forcefully, it is impossible to remove all the air from the lungs, and this volume that remains is called the residual volume.

The digestive system

104. A Prehension is the term that means to pick up food

Deglutition describes swallowing.

Peristalsis refers to the waves of smooth muscle contraction which push the bolus of food through the digestive tract.

Egestion is the evacuation of the waste products left in the digestive tract after digestion and absorption. Defaecation refers to the same process!

105. B The philtrum is the cleft in the upper lip

The corner of the mouth can be referred to as the commissure of the lips. The piece of tissue found under the tongue is the frenulum, and the technical term for the gums is the gingiva.

106. C The dog has four pairs of salivary glands

The four pairs of glands are the sublingual, submandibular (also called mandibular), parotid and zygomatic salivary glands.

107. C The correct dental formula for a kitten is I 3/3 C 1/1 PM 3/2

The dental formulae shown are all correct for cats and dogs at different stages of their development

I 3/3 C 1/1 PM 3/3 is the formula for the deciduous teeth of a dog

I 3/3 C 1/1 PM 4/4 M 2/3 is the formula for the adult dentition of the dog

I 3/3 C 1/1 PM 3/2 M 1/1 is the dental formula for an adult cat

108. B The region of the stomach closest to the oesophagus is the cardia

The oesophagus joins the stomach at the cardiac sphincter, a weak sphincter which helps to prevent food returning from the stomach into the oesophagus.

The main section of the stomach is the fundus. The stomach is C-shaped; the outer side of the C is referred to as the greater curvature, and the inside is the lesser curvature.

The junction between the stomach and small intestine is the pyloric sphincter. This is much stronger than the cardiac sphincter, and food is unable to enter the small intestine until it is of the correct consistency.

109. A The double fold of peritoneum that links the stomach to the abdominal wall is called the omentum

Mesentery is similar, except that this links the intestines to the wall. Ligaments are also double layers of peritoneum – for example the broad ligament which extends from the uterus. The term serosa is used more generally to indicate the peritoneal covering of any abdominal organ.

110. C Parietal cells in the stomach wall secrete hydrochloric acid

Three of the cells listed are found in the stomach, and these are all found in gastric pits.

Goblet cells secrete mucus, parietal cells secrete acid, and chief cells secrete pepsinogen which is then converted into the enzyme pepsin.

Beta cells are not found in the stomach, but are important secretory cells in the pancreas, where they produce insulin.

111. C The gall bladder empties into the duodenum

Bile produced by the liver is secreted into the duodenum in response to the hormone secretin. This is needed for the digestion of fats.

112. A Chyle is contained within the lacteals

Chyle is the name of the fluid that forms within the lacteals, which are part of the lymphatic system. Chyle consists of fluid collected from the interstitial spaces and some nutrients including fatty acids, which give chyle its milky appearance.

Answers

Chyme is the name of the partially digested food that leaves the stomach and enters the small intestine.

Bile is needed to help with fat digestion, and is produced by the liver and stored in the gall bladder until needed. It is then released into the duodenum via the common bile duct.

Proteins are digested, and then absorbed from the intestine directly into the blood capillaries before being taken to the liver via the hepatic portal vein.

113. B   The enzyme that breaks down proteins in the small intestine is trypsin

Trypsin is a protease secreted by the pancreas in pancreatic juice. Pepsin is also a protease, but is secreted in the stomach, where it works best under acid conditions. This becomes less active when pH conditions change to alkaline as the food enters the small intestine.

Amylases break down carbohydrates, and lipases digest fats.

114. A   The section of the intestine that absorbs water in the dog and cat is the colon

The colon is the longest section of the large intestine, and its main role is the absorption of water and electrolytes from its lumen. The caecum is a blind-ending sac (the appendix in humans), which has very little function in carnivores. In herbivores this may be well-developed as a site for bacterial fermentation.

The jejunum and ileum are both sections of the small intestine, and both are involved in the absorption of nutrients other than water. There is also some digestion still taking place within the jejunum.

115. B   Synthesis of vitamins, including vitamins A and D, is not a function of the liver

Although the liver is involved in the storage of the fat-soluble vitamins, which include A and D, it does not synthesise them, or there would be no dietary requirement for these.

The liver is, however, very important, and carries out a

range of functions including fat metabolism, deamination of amino acids and the destruction of old red blood cells.

Other roles include the synthesis of plasma proteins, bile formation, carbohydrate metabolism, iron storage, thermoregulation and detoxification/deactivation of various chemicals and hormones.

The urinary system

116. C   The glomeruli are located in the renal cortex

A glomerulus is a network of capillaries, and this is where filtration of the blood takes place, and the filtrate (the fluid that will be modified to form urine) is collected in the glomerular capsule or Bowman's capsule.

The outermost part of the kidney is the capsule, made of irregular dense connective tissue. Underneath this is the vascular cortex. The medulla lies more centrally and this is where the loops of Henle and the collecting ducts are found. The renal pelvis is where the urine collects before leaving the kidney via the ureter.

117. B   The indentation on the side of the kidney where the renal blood vessels and the ureter emerge is called the hilus

The calyx is the area the urine flows through as it collects in the renal pelvis before going into the ureter.

The renal pyramids are triangular areas of tissue where the collecting ducts are found. The point of each triangle or pyramid is referred to as the apex.

118. D   The correct order is proximal convoluted tubule, loop of Henle, distal convoluted tubule, collecting duct

119. A   Sodium is only reabsorbed by the distal convoluted tubule if aldosterone is present

Without the presence of aldosterone, the urine's electrolyte content is not altered at this site.

The other three hormones listed all have links with renal function. Renin and erythropoietin are both produced by the kidney. Erythropoietin stimulates red blood cell maturation. Renin stimulates the conversion of angiotensinogen in the plasma to the active form angiotensin. This then acts on blood vessels causing vasoconstriction, and on the adrenal cortex to stimulate the release of aldosterone.

120. D Anti-diuretic hormone is produced by the posterior pituitary

ADH acts on the renal tubules and causes the wall of the collecting duct in particular to become permeable to water. The high salt concentrations within the medulla draw water out of the renal tubule, and the urine becomes more concentrated.

121. D The unusual property of transitional epithelium compared with other epithelia is that it is able to stretch

Transitional epithelium is a stratified epithelium. This means that the cells are layered on top of each other, which means that it is impermeable. This is not unique to transitional epithelium; for example, the squamous epithelium which forms the epidermis is also stratified.

Whilst the epithelium is able to stretch, it does not totally contract down around a tear. This would be a very useful property – animals with ruptured bladders would be considerably less at risk from uraemia and peritonitis, but alas this is not the case!

122. B The kidney secretes the hormone renin if there is low blood pressure

Renin is secreted by the kidney in response to falling arterial blood pressure, since if this happens, less blood will be filtered, and urea and other waste products will not be removed from the body.

The renin converts inactive angiotensinogen in the bloodstream into the active form, angiotensin, which causes vasoconstriction, thereby increasing blood pressure.

Angiotensin also stimulates the production of aldosterone by the adrenal cortex, and this causes sodium to be reabsorbed by the body, particularly from the distal convoluted tubule. This has an osmotic effect, drawing with it water, and so this too acts to increase the circulating blood volume, and improve blood pressure.

123. C Urine flow along the ureter to the bladder is driven by peristaltic contractions of smooth muscle

124. C **The statement that sympathetic neurons are involved in the process of micturition and stimulate bladder contraction is untrue.**

The bladder has two sphincters as stated. The inner one is made of smooth muscle, and under parasympathetic stimulation this relaxes, and the muscle wall of the bladder starts to contract. Around the outside of this is a second sphincter made of skeletal muscle, which is under voluntary or somatic control.

The nerves that supply the bladder and the rest of the caudal pelvis are the sacral spinal nerves. Sympathetic neurons are not directly involved in the response.

The reproductive system

125. C Spermatozoa are produced in the seminiferous tubules

The seminiferous tubules are found within the testes. The sperm are produced here; they then move into the efferent tubules before collecting within the epididymis. The deferent duct then leads from the epididymis to the urethra.

126. A The cells of Leydig produce the hormone testosterone

Testosterone is needed to stimulate sperm production and for generation of secondary sex characteristics. The sperm are actually produced by spermatogenic cells or spermatogonia. A third type of cell, the Sertoli cell, produces nutrients for the spermatozoa and also produces oestrogen.

127. D The efferent tubule does not form part of the spermatic cord.

The spermatic cord is made of all the structures that run from the abdominal cavity to the scrotum, and it includes the tunica vaginalis (vaginal tunic), the deferent duct, the cremaster muscle, the spermatic artery and vein, and the spermatic nerve. The efferent tubules are found within the structure of the testis, and link the seminiferous tubules to the epididymis.

128. C The seminal fluid produced by accessory glands in the male does not carry enzymes needed for fertilisation

The spermatozoa all have enzymes within the acrosome in the 'head' of the sperm. Therefore there is no need for any further enzyme assistance from the seminal fluid.

All the other statements are functions of this fluid.

129. B It is untrue that the os penis only develops in the dog, and does not form in the cat

Both species have an os penis. The only difference is that the bone does not always fully ossify in the cat, and may not show up well on radiographs, whereas it always does in the dog. The other statements are all true.

130. B A female animal pregnant with her first litter can be described as primigravid

An animal, such as man, which normally bears one offspring at a time is described as uniparous; those that bear several young are multiparous. Whenever an animal enters her natural breeding time, she can either enter oestrus just once (as the bitch does) in which case she is described as monoestrous, or she might enter oestrus more than once (like the queen), in which case she is polyoestrous.

131. D Luteinising hormone is needed to trigger ovulation

The four hormones listed are all needed for completion of the oestrous cycle. Follicle stimulating hormone is released by the pituitary, and this causes the follicles to mature within the ovary. They release oestrogen which gives rise to the physical and behavioural signs seen during pro-oestrus and oestrus. Luteinising hormone is only released when oestrogen levels are high, and this causes ovulation. The structure remaining within the ovary, the corpus luteum, produces progesterone, needed for the maintenance of pregnancy.

132. B The section of the broad ligament which lies over the uterine tube or oviduct is the mesosalpinx

The broad ligament is a double fold of peritoneum that links the female reproductive tract to the body wall. It is divided into parts associated with the ovary – the mesovarium, the uterine tube – the mesosalpinx and the uterus itself, the mesometrium. The mesoureter is another fold of peritoneum which covers the ureter.

133. A Progesterone is the hormone that always has an inhibitory effect on the release of follicle stimulating hormone

Progesterone is released by the corpus luteum, and prepares the uterus for possible pregnancy. It also inhibits the release of gonadotrophin releasing hormone (GRH) by the hypothalamus which is needed to trigger FSH production. Oestrogen also may influence FSH production. At low levels it indicates that the follicles which produce it are developing, but are not yet mature. As they grow the amount of oestrogen released increases, and when it reaches maximal amounts, this exerts a feedback effect on the pituitary such that no more FSH is produced, and luteinising hormone is released instead. This causes ovulation to take place.

134. C   The infundibulum is found at the proximal end of the uterine tube (oviduct)

The infundibulum is the opening into the uterine tube. This is where the ova enter the uterine tube after their release from the ovary. The ova are helped by finger-like projections at the edge of the opening called fimbriae, which waft the eggs into the centre of the infundibulum and on into the uterine tube.

135. D   The external urethral orifice is located in the floor of the vagina

The external urethral orifice is the opening of the urethra, and is the point where the urinary and genital systems join. It marks the boundary between the vagina and the vestibule – the vestibule being the area caudal to the opening which leads to the vulval lips.

136. B   The cervix is only open during oestrus

Normally the cervix is tightly closed, but during oestrus it relaxes slightly to allow the sperm through if the animal has been mated. After oestrus, neutrophils are produced to clear the area of any possible infection before the cervix closes once again.

137. B   The queen is a seasonal breeder

The queen is an induced ovulator, and without mating she will not ovulate and will therefore not enter metoestrus.

She is also polyoestrous, rather than monoestrous, since she will enter oestrus several times within one breeding season. The duration of oestrus is slightly variable depending on whether the queen is mated or not, but usually she calls for about 3-6 days if mated, 5-10 days if not.

138. C False pregnancy often develops during metoestrus in the bitch

Metoestrus is the stage that is dominated by the presence of the corpus luteum which produces progesterone. In most species this period is quite short and the corpus luteum regresses, but in the bitch the corpus luteum remains viable for much longer, almost mimicking the duration of pregnancy. This predisposes the bitch to developing the signs of false pregnancy, such as nest building, mothering behaviour with toys, and even milk production.

139. B Mammary glands are modified apocrine glands

Apocrine glands are basically sweat glands, and these are found all over the body. Mammary glands are modified apocrine glands, so although the secretion is not the same as sweat, it is still a water-based secretion.

Merocrine glands are a slightly different type of sweat gland found only on the pads of the feet.

Sebaceous glands produce sebum, an oily secretion needed to maintain the quality of the hair coat.

Endocrine glands secrete hormones directly into the bloodstream. All the other glands mentioned in this question are exocrine glands – where the secretions act locally and are delivered to the skin surface via ducts.

140. A A zygote is a fertilised ovum

Once an ovum is fertilised it can either be called a zygote or conceptus. This then starts dividing to form a ball of cells which develop a fluid-filled space in the middle. It is then called a blastocyst, and it implants in the wall of the uterine horn. Next the inner cell mass within the blastocyst starts to differentiate and forms the embryo. The embryos of many species appear the same initially, but once recognisable features develop (usually about 35 days in the dog and cat) it can be called a foetus.

141. C   Implantation of the blastocysts takes place 14-20 days after ovulation in the bitch

142. B   The fluid-filled sac which lies closest to the foetus and protects it during delivery is the amnion

The allantois initially contains waste products from the developing embryo. Later, part of it forms the placenta as the allantoic membrane merges with a second membrane, the chorion, and villi form between this and the uterine wall.

The yolk sac is a temporary structure, and this provides nutrients in the early stages of embryonic development before the placenta is formed. This has completely disappeared before birth.

143. A   Cats and dogs have a zonary placenta

The placenta forms a band all the way round the embryonic membranes in animals which have a zonary placenta.

Other species, however, do differ in the type of placenta used. For example primates have a discoid placenta, and sheep have a cotyledonous placenta.

The Integument

144. D **The cells in the stratum corneum layer of the skin are those that have no nuclei and are fully keratinised.**

The base layer of the epidermis is where the cells divide, and this is the stratum basale or stratum germinativum.

The layer above this is the stratum granulosum, where the cells are slightly more flattened, and where the keratin starts to be deposited. It is in the next layer that the cells lose their nuclei – the stratum lucidum.

145. A **Merocrine glands are only found on the pads of the feet**

There are two types of sweat glands in the skin – apocrine glands which are found all over the skin, and merocrine glands found specifically in the footpads. These secrete watery secretions.

Sebaceous glands produce a more oily secretion, sebum, which helps to give the hair coat its natural sheen, and to provide a degree of water-proofing. Sebaceous glands are therefore found in close association with the hairs of the body, and there are particularly high numbers of these glands along the spinal ridge of animals.

Meibomian glands are a type of sebaceous gland found only in the eye. They produce a secretion needed to lubricate and protect the cornea.

146. D **Grooming does not influence the moulting of the hair coat**

Moulting is naturally related to the season, with animals tending to shed more hair in the transition from winter to summer, and vice versa. However, this may be less noticeable in animals housed indoors due to the effects of central heating and artificial lighting. Hormones also play a role – thyroid hormones are needed to start the hair growth cycle, but steroid hormones can inhibit the production of new hair growth. Therefore hormone imbalances may lead to the development of alopecia. This is usually bilaterally symmetrical and often seen along the flank of the animal.

Grooming does not actually alter the hair growth cycle, but is a useful way of ensuring that dead fur is removed, and that the animal does not ingest too much fur. Animals which are not groomed, may develop *trichobezoars* or fur balls.

147. A The type of hair attached to the arrector pili muscle is guard hair

Guard hairs or primary hairs form the coarse outer coat. Beneath this lie the wool hairs or secondary hairs which provide the insulating undercoat. It is only the guard hairs that can be raised, and once raised they trap a thicker layer of air against the animal's skin which acts as an insulator and reduces heat loss.

The vibrissae are whiskers, and these are mostly found on the animal's face. They have far more sensory nerve endings associated with the hair papilla than other hair types, and provide the animal with tactile cues about its environment. They are also the first hairs to develop in the foetus.

148. D There are seven pads on each forelimb of a cat.

There are five digital pads, four next to the main digits, and one adjacent to the dewclaw. There is a central pad, or metacarpal pad, and the carpal or 'stopper' pad.

149. B Cat claws are held in the retracted position by elastic ligaments

However, when the cat wishes to use its claws, contraction of the digital flexors causes the claws to become unsheathed.

2 Observation and care of the patient

1. A   **It would be inappropriate to place a male dog in close proximity to a bitch in season**

This would be stressful for both in-patients. Pheromones and hormone-linked behaviours would make both animals very agitated since the urge to mate would be very strong.

The other statements relating to the care of hospitalised patients are all good practical advice – the advice about urination and defaecation being particularly important, bearing in mind that different animals may have different toileting preferences. This may relate to the type of surface on which they are expected to toilet or to the degree of privacy.

2. D   **The case that should give you cause for concern is the dog with a temperature of 103°F or 39.4°C**

This temperature is outside the normal range, and this should be checked against the reason for the dog's hospitalisation, and any other temperature readings already taken. It should be recorded, and if markedly different from that expected or from previous readings, the vet should be informed.

Capillary refill times of healthy animals are normally less than 2 seconds, so a CRT of 1 second is quite acceptable.

Rabbits' urine is very variable in colour, and can be quite yellow, but can vary through the spectrum to a very dark red colour. This should be noted, but is not necessarily abnormal.

Many cats resent being hospitalised, and may well be disinterested in food. If this is very different behaviour from that shown before, then it would be a concern, but for many animals this is their normal reaction to a situation they find stressful. Monitor these animals closely – it may be necessary to think of alternative ways to make them feel more relaxed so that they are able to eat.

3. A   The term pica means a depraved appetite

Pica can take a number of forms, and different species may show different eating behaviours. Coprophagy in dogs may be considered abnormal, though of course this would be quite appropriate for a rabbit, for example.

Anorexia means absence of appetite and no desire to eat.

Dysphagia refers to difficulty eating. This could be due to pain in the oral cavity or some type of physical problem making eating more problematic for the animal.

4. B   The normal urine output for a dog is 1-2 ml/kg/hour

Often urine outputs are quoted as around 20 ml/kg/day. This is fine as a general rule of thumb, but for hospitalised patients it is easier to measure output over a shorter period of time. Urine output is likely to be higher in animals on drips than otherwise, and this should always be taken into consideration.

5. D   A cream vaginal discharge is always abnormal

Cream-coloured discharges usually only develop when there is some type of bacterial infection present. It is impossible to state from the discharge where the source of the problem might be – it could be a vaginitis, or it could be a metritis or even a pyometra. Further investigation would be required.

A bloody discharge could be abnormal, but this is also seen in a bitch in pro-oestrus. As she approaches oestrus the amount of blood reduces, and the discharge becomes more straw coloured.

Dark green/brown discharges are often seen at the time of parturition. This is due to blood breakdown products being released as the placentae separate from the uterine wall.

6. C   Petechiae might be seen in an animal with a bleeding disorder

Petechiae are small pin-point haemorrhages which may be visible on the surface of non-pigmented mucous membranes.

An anaemic animal would show pale mucous membranes; an animal with respiratory obstruction is likely to show cyanotic or blue mucous membranes and the jaundiced animal would appear yellow.

7. B   The correct formula for the conversion of temperature from degrees Fahrenheit to degrees Centigrade is (°F – 32) x 5 ÷ 9

To change the temperature from degrees Centigrade to degrees Fahrenheit the formula is (°C x 9 ÷ 5) + 32

8. C   The alternative to using the rectal route to take a temperature is to use the external ear canal

However, it should be noted that normal temperatures will be about 2°C cooler than the equivalent rectal reading. Another site that could be used is the axilla, or armpit, and the same consideration should be made.

The forehead and sublingual areas are not suitable in animals, despite being used extensively in humans, the reasons being that the fur prevents an accurate forehead temperature being read and an animal might chew a thermometer placed sublingually.

Between the digits is also unsuitable since this is too peripheral and would vary with environmental temperature rather than reflecting core body temperature.

9. C   Respirations should be counted for 1 minute in order to determine respiratory rate

10. B   Ectothermic means the same as poikilothermic

An ectothermic or poikilothermic animal is one which is
unable to regulate its own body temperature fully, and is
dependent on environmental heat to keep itself warm
enough to function normally.

**11. D   All the methods listed are useful in the prevention of
decubitus ulcers**

Decubitus ulcers are pressure sores, caused by an animal
remaining in one position for long periods of time. They are
most common over bony areas such as the elbows and
greater trochanters of the hip region.

**12. C   A petroleum jelly impregnated gauze dressing would be
most appropriate to use for a burn**

Burns and scalds often cause marked damage to the
epidermis which exposes the vascular dermis beneath. It is
important that this tissue does not dry out, so gauze
dressings impregnated with petroleum jelly are useful,
acting as a barrier to evaporation of water.

The other dressings would all stick to the dermis, and cause
damage when removed.

13. A   A Velpeau sling should be used after a shoulder luxation

This type of bandage is used to immobilise the foreleg with
the shoulder, elbow and carpal joints held in a flexed
position. It prevents the animal from weight bearing and
therefore allows time for the shoulder joint to settle down
first.

**14. A   Medicines take longest to be effective if given via the
oral route**

There can also be variation in how well individual patients
absorb the specific drugs given. Usually it is expected that a
drug would take over an hour to take effect if given this
way.

15. D   Heat should be applied in the case of an abscess

Heat can be helpful in this situation since it draws the pus to a head, and stimulates the local blood supply which brings white blood cells to the area to help fight the infection.

16. B   It takes about 20-30 minutes for intramuscular injections to take effect

The times suggested refer to the major routes of drug administration – thus 30-45 minutes would be the time expected for subcutaneous injections, 0-2 minutes for intravenous injections and over an hour for oral treatments.

17. D   The lumbodorsal muscles can be used as a site for the administration of intramuscular injections

The gluteals and hamstrings muscles should be avoided due to the risk of injuring the sciatic nerve. The anterior tibial is a very small muscle running down the front of the tibia, and it would be easy to hit the bone beneath and cause pain.

18. A   The top of vials containing hormones should never be wiped with an alcohol swab

Alcohol is a disinfectant, and it acts by causing proteins to denature. Several of the hormones are proteins, for example insulin, and there is therefore a risk that the alcohol may come into contact with the hormone preparation and inactivate it.

3 First aid

1. B   **The word triage refers to the prioritising of cases for treatment**

2. C   **The most important assessment to make when dealing with an emergency patient is whether it has a patent airway or not**

Airway obstruction is the fastest way in which a patient may die, and so this must be the first thing to check.

Breathing is next, followed by circulation. Checking the circulation usually involves checking for a pulse and making an assessment of the colour of the mucous membranes and capillary refill time.

Shock and haemorrhage are both potentially life threatening, but usually dealt with after the A,B,C have been checked and found to be adequate.

3. C   **It is incorrect that other than an animal stretcher, a blanket is the best form of stretcher to use**

Blankets are readily available, and are therefore often used, but the main problem with these is that the animal is not well supported. It usually ends up in a heap in the middle of the blanket. This would therefore be particularly dangerous if spinal injuries were suspected. A more rigid stretcher should be improvised – this could be a solid piece of wood, or a stretcher made out of broom handles and a buttoned coat with the sleeves turned inside out, so that the poles could be slid through these.

4. C   **The term strabismus means a squint**

Two of the other conditions listed also have specific names. Nystagmus is used to describe the flickering of the eyes, and anisocoria means that the pupil sizes are not the same.

5. D **Decreased capillary refill time is not a sign seen in shock**

Normal capillary refill time is usually under 2 seconds, but in shock this may well increase to over 3 seconds, suggesting that the peripheral circulation is very poor. This ties in with the extremities being cold, and the mucous membranes appearing pale.

Shock is a state of circulatory collapse, so the heart tries to compensate by speeding up, but this does not always help. Respiration is also usually increased in an attempt to improve the oxygenation of the tissues.

6. B **It might be appropriate to use a hypertonic solution intravenously if an animal has had a head injury leading to compression of the brain**

In this type of case the inflammatory response causes the brain to swell, and this makes the compression even worse. This will ultimately lead to the death of the nerve cells. Hypertonic solutions can be used to draw fluid out of cells and away from the interstitial spaces, and therefore reduce the swelling of the brain tissue.

7. D **The correct resuscitation protocol is to give 2 breaths every 15 cardiac compressions**

This, incidentally, is the same as is recommended for an adult human patient.

8. A **A cat might show hindlimb paralysis with cold toes if it was suffering from arterial thromboembolism**

This condition arises when a blood clot lodges within a major vessel. One of the common sites of occurrence is at the division of the aorta where it splits into the internal and external iliac arteries. The tissues supplied by the blocked vessels become cold to the touch and are unable to function normally.

9. B   **The animal that should be seen by a vet as soon as possible is the bitch that has shown a green-brown discharge without any other signs of starting to whelp**

All the other situations described could be quite normal, therefore although these animals should be monitored closely throughout their parturition, they do not need to be seen immediately.

10. D   **It would be inappropriate to try to resuscitate a neonate by intermittent positive pressure ventilation using an anaesthetic circuit and oxygen**

In order to ventilate an animal efficiently on an anaesthetic circuit, it would need to be intubated. It might prove very difficult to find tubes of a suitable size quickly enough, and time would be wasted trying to intubate the neonate.

All the other techniques will help and can be carried out quickly.

11. A   **Hypocalcaemia seen in pregnancy or lactation is also referred to as eclampsia**

Paraphimosis is the name given to the condition in which a male animal is unable to retract its penis into the prepuce.

Pyometra is a potentially life-threatening condition in which the uterus becomes infected, and full of pus.

Pseudocyesis is an alternative name for false pregnancy.

12. C   **The advice that would be inappropriate to give the owner of a fitting dog would be to ensure that its tongue is pulled forward**

Whilst it would be very helpful in preventing the animal choking on its tongue, it is too dangerous to suggest that an owner tries this. The dog is not conscious and therefore not in control of its actions, and is quite likely to accidentally bite the owner.

Darkening and quietening the room is very useful since this reduces external stimuli that might encourage the dog to keep fitting. It is also useful to move objects away from the dog so that it does not hurt itself on these.

13. A **The condition that might result in an animal showing pollakiuria is cystitis**

Pollakiuria describes the passing of small amounts of urine frequently. This is a common finding in animals with cystitis, which feel the need to pass urine due to the inflammation of the bladder, although there is very little urine actually present.

14. A **The disease condition that should be suspected in a collapsed animal with a sweet smell on its breath is diabetes mellitus**

In the last stages of diabetes mellitus, ketones build up within the circulation. These cause neurological signs since they are toxic, and the animals may collapse and lose consciousness. Ketones have a characteristic sweet odour, and this may be smelt on the breath. The other conditions listed can also lead to collapse, but in none of these would a sweet smell be detected.

However, it is important to note that not everyone can smell ketones, and if you are one of these people then you should not rule out the possibility of a collapsed animal having diabetes mellitus just because you cannot smell it.

15. C **The condition that could be life threatening is a bee sting**

Bee stings can vary in severity from something that is irritating and uncomfortable to the animal, to something that could cause death. This is mainly due to the location of the sting – stings to the pharynx can cause sufficient swelling to obstruct the airway, whereas more superficial stings are not usually a problem. The other situation in which stings can be life threatening is if an animal suffers an anaphylactic reaction. Advice should always be given to owners as to what to watch out for so that help can be given as soon as necessary.

16. B   The first action that should be taken if an animal is suspected of having ingested paraquat is to induce emesis

Paraquat is a very dangerous poison and can be lethal. It initially damages the kidneys, and can cause death through renal failure. If the animal survives this, then it is still likely to die since the alveolar walls in the lungs become thickened, and the animal eventually is unable to breath adequately. This is quite protracted, and takes about 10 days to develop. Therefore the most important course of action to take is to induce vomiting as soon after ingestion as possible. Fuller's earth may then be given to try to prevent absorption of the poison. After that supportive treatments should be given, but owners should be warned of the poor prognosis.

17. C   Appropriate treatment for acute paraphimosis would be irrigation with cold water

Paraphimosis is the inability to retract a protruding penis. By cooling the area with cold water it should encourage the swelling to reduce, and with assistance the penis should be replaceable. Ice packs would not be a good idea, since the tissue may suffer cold burns, and this could lead to longterm damage to the penis.

18. A   The poison that can cause central blindness is lead

The other poisons may all lead to neurological signs, but the only one that prevents the animal from seeing whilst conscious is lead.

19. A   The body deals with haemorrhage in a number of ways, but this does not involve the production of inflammatory mediators

Chemicals such as histamine are released when tissues are damaged, and they induce an inflammatory response. This actually increases the amount of haemorrhage from a wound since the chemicals cause vasodilation which increases blood flow to the area.

20. D **The best action to take initially is to apply indirect pressure**

If there is a suspicion that there is a foreign body in a wound, then direct pressure should be avoided, since although it is a very good technique for reducing and controlling haemorrhage, it would also push any foreign body further into the tissues.

The brachial pressure point can be useful to control haemorrhage in the foreleg distal to the mid-humerus, but would not be much use for a wound in the back leg!

Tourniquets are occasionally used, but should only be used as a last resort since they have to be applied tightly enough to occlude both arteries and veins, and therefore cut off the entire blood supply to the limb. They should be used for a maximum of about 10 minutes before slowly releasing the tourniquet to allow fresh blood to the tissues.

21. C **Burns caused by extreme cold are usually the slowest to show the severity of the damage caused.**

Dry heat will show damage at the time of injury, but burns due to hot fats or steam may take a little longer to show since the fur may not be burnt away at the time of the incident. The fur will take a few days to fall out, and then the extent of the skin damage will be visible.

22. A **It is contraindicated to use a concentrated salt solution to induce emesis**

In many cases it simply does not work, which means that the toxin is still active, and worse still, the animal's electrolyte balance may be seriously affected.

Mustard solutions are also not terribly effective, but do not do any harm, so can be used as a last resort.

Washing soda crystals and apomorphine both work well, though note that the latter, being a prescription drug, should only be given under the direction of a veterinary surgeon.

23. D   A fracture in which there are several fracture fragments is described as comminuted

Multiple fractures describe a situation when there is more than one fracture site. Complicated fractures are those in which some other structure has also been damaged, for example a nerve or major blood vessel.

A compound fracture, or open fracture, has a wound overlying the fracture site. This can provide access for bacteria, and care must be taken to clean the wounds as thoroughly as possible before repair is attempted.

24. C   The first aid management for a luxation is to restrict movement of the affected joint

A luxation is simply a dislocation of two bones forming a joint. No attempt should be made to reduce the dislocation, since this is likely to be extremely painful. It could also result in the worsening of some types of luxation.

Rest is essential, and if the animal will tolerate it, a support bandage is helpful. Cold compresses can also be used to reduce swelling at the site.

4 Animal handling and basic animal management

1. C   **A rolled up towel can be used to restrain the head of a brachycephalic dog**

This can be a useful technique for dealing with small brachycephalics, since it is often impossible to use muzzles in these breeds.

It may be possible to restrain some cats with the use of a cat muzzle that not only stops the cat being able to bite easily, but also covers the eyes. However other animals will panic even more, and this will make them very difficult to control.

Rabbits should never be handled by the ears. The scruff can be used, but only if the hindquarters of the animal are supported properly. Similarly it is inappropriate to use the tail to lift a rat. Most rats tolerate being held around the thorax with the hindquarters supported.

2. A   **A dog catcher should only be used as a last resort when restraining a dog.**

The use of a dog catcher is often very traumatic for dogs handled this way, so other methods should be attempted first.

The basket type muzzles can be very effective at preventing animals from being able to bite providing they are used correctly.

Tape muzzles are a useful improvised way of preventing dogs from biting in an emergency. However, it is important that the tape is tied tightly enough and this may cause pain and bruising to the muzzle

3. C   **You should still be wary of a dog wagging its tail since nervous or aggressive dogs may show this**

Many happy animals will greet humans by wagging the tail, showing an intention to please. However, nervous dogs may use the same signal as a sign of appeasement, and in aggressive animals it may be interpreted as an intention to interact – probably aggressively.

4. B   **You should avoid making prolonged eye contact as you approach a nervous dog**

It is important to appreciate from the dog's perspective how you appear as you approach the animal; if you rush the animal or approach it before it is ready, it is likely to judge this as being aggressive, and will therefore prepare to defend itself. Open hands can be seen as weapons, or as an easy appendage to attack, and prolonged eye contact may be seen as a challenge to which the dog is likely to respond.

5. D   **If a dog growls at you, the best course of action to take is to muzzle it**

In this situation it is worth taking the time to muzzle the dog with a good basket style muzzle. This will ensure that if the growl is a prelude to attack, you will not be harmed. However, if it was just a warning, then no harm has come to the animal.

The other courses of action suggested could all encourage the dog to carry on growling or may even lead it to attack, since all may reinforce the unwanted behaviour. Comfort may act as a reward, punishment justifies the dog's approach, and backing off proves to the dog that its growling was effective.

6. C   **It is never safe to leave a dog with a choke chain with a lead attached**

There is a strong possibility that the dog could do itself considerable harm by pulling against the lead, and strangulation has been known to occur with this type of method.

All of the other methods can be used. If there is space

available, a long lead can be used to tie an animal outside a kennel. Choke chains should not be used in this instance either.

If the second method is used, leaving the end of the lead outside the kennel, then it is very important that the animal is supervised carefully to avoid the risk of strangulation.

For some animals the best technique, rather than trying to go into the kennel to get the dog out, is to ensure that the kennel area is clear of other animals and the door is closed, and then open the kennel door, and stand to one side of the door to give the dog a clear view. Then as it comes forward a slip lead can be placed over the dog's head. Once a lead is in place, these animals will usually walk out without further incident.

7. A **The minimum and maximum temperatures recommended for boarding kennels are 10°C – 26°C**

8. C **The minimum recommended height for a unit within a boarding cattery is 1.8 m (6 ft)**

9. A **Ventilation bricks can be used to provide a system of passive ventilation**

Active ventilation systems all require the use of fans or air-conditioning units. Insulation is useful to help reduce heat losses, but does not contribute to the air changes that are required to prevent the build up of ammonia, humidity and organisms.

10. A **A biguanide can be used to cleanse wounds**

These include products such as chlorhexidine, which have low toxicity and irritancy. Even though they are relatively non-toxic, it is still important that a dilute solution is used (0.5%), since more concentrated solutions could cause some tissue damage in open wounds.

These compounds can also be referred to as diguanides.

11. C   Chloroxylenol is a phenolic disinfectant

There are several different types of phenolic disinfectants, and chloroxylenol is a synthetic chlorinated phenol. It is not suitable for skin disinfection in animals, but can be used in the environment. Also the phenolics often have quite pungent odours, which may not be appreciated by the animals!

Glutaraldehyde is an aldehyde, and the halogenated tertiary amines and povidone-iodine both come under the halogen grouping.

12. B   Quaternary ammonium compounds act as cationic surfactants

A surfactant can be described as a 'wetting compound' since it acts to reduce the surface tension of aqueous solutions. Some are weak disinfectants, such as cetrimide, whereas others have no disinfectant properties. However, if they are mixed with other suitable disinfectants, they may increase the penetrating power of the solution and achieve a more effective kill of the micro-organisms.

13. C   It is not true that short-coated animals do not need to be groomed

All the other statements are true. The only animals that may not be groomed during their stay are as follows:

• Very short stay patients
• Patients with conditions that would be worsened by grooming
• Patients with very aggressive temperaments – this would increase stress levels for both patient and nurse, and if not needed for medical reasons is perhaps best left undone.

14. C   It is useful to use finger stall toothbrushes as a means of introducing an animal to the sensation of bristles

However, a careful assessment of the animal's temperament should be made before this is attempted!

Once the finger stall brush is accepted then a special animal toothbrush can be used. These are different from human ones, since the size of the head and handle have been adapted to match the oral cavity of the species for which they are intended. It is also important to use animal toothpastes. Human toothpaste can lead to fluoride toxicity in animals, and there may be resentment due to the strong flavours we like.

Mouthwashes can be used, but these are usually just breath fresheners, since animals don't usually 'swoosh' the liquid around their mouth sufficiently to give antibacterial protection. Therefore they are not suitable to use in place of brushing.

15. C   A styptic is used to control mild haemorrhage

There are a number of substances that can be used as styptics including silver nitrate pencils, potassium permanganate, ferric chloride and friar's balsam. The most common reason for their use is if the quick is accidentally cut whilst trimming an animal's claws.

16. B   The quarantine period for animals entering the UK that are not covered by the PETS scheme is six months

17. C   It is not necessary for animals to be tattooed with permanent identification

Animals must be microchipped to provide definitive identification of the animal. Tattooing is not acceptable.

The other statements about the scheme are quite correct.

18. A   Primates are not exempt from quarantine

The requirements for any unusual species or wild animal should be checked before any attempt is made to bring the animal into the country. It is best to contact DEFRA for details.

19. D   All of the dogs named are prohibited under the Dangerous Dogs Act 1991 with the exception of the Dogue de Bordeaux

The Dogue de Bordeaux is a mastiff type of dog, but is not

named as a dangerous dog – most in fact are gentle giants! The fourth breed specifically mentioned in the Act is the Fila Braziliero.

All the breeds named are dogs that have been bred for fighting, and are therefore considered to have too many dangerous traits in their genetic make-up.

20. B   The organisation that recognises and classifies pedigree cat breeds in the UK is the Governing Council of Cat Fancy (GCCF)

The Feline Advisory Bureau is a charity involved in feline welfare, which also funds research to benefit cats. The other organisations suggested do not actually exist.

21. B   A hound glove would be suitable for use on a short-coated breed of dog

The other pieces of equipment are more suited to animals with either longer coats, or dense undercoats.

22. A   The group recognised by the Kennel Club that is classed as Non-sporting is the Working group

The seven groups recognised by the Kennel Club are divided as follows:

- *Sporting*
  1. Hound group
  2. Gundog group
  3. Terrier group
- *Non-sporting*
  1. Utility group
  2. Pastoral group
  3. Working group
  4. Toy group

5 Practice organisation, management, law and ethics

1. A   **A written statement of a business's purpose is its mission statement**

The mission statement simply sets out the basic principles to which the business intends to adhere. ˙

Business plans set out in precise detail objectives for a given period of time, such as 3-5 years, and looks at how the objectives will be achieved.

A financial plan is less concerned with the 'how', but sets out the costs involved, and matches this against projected income for the period described in the business plan.

SWOT analyses can be carried out for almost anything, but are a very useful tool in determining what stage a business has reached. SWOT is an acronym for the 4 areas to be considered – strengths, weaknesses, opportunities and threats.

2. C   **The statement that more clients are lost as a result of their animal dying at the surgery than due to poor communication skills of veterinary staff is untrue**

It is likely that a client given incorrect or inappropriate information, or treated in an off-hand manner, will leave a practice. Often the association is that if communication is careless at a particular surgery, then the attention the animal receives would also be shoddy. However, the death of an animal at the surgery, if handled sensitively, does not automatically mean the client feels a bad job has been done, and in some cases, the care shown to the client will actually lead them to recommend the surgery to other potential clients.

3. D   **It is true that practices must keep employee PAYE records for at least 3 years**

Clients and employees have a statutory right to access any records that are held about them by practices.

Practices which keep computerised records about clients, animals and employees should be registered with the Data Protection Registrar, so that individuals whose details are kept this way are protected. This does not apply to written records.

There is no legally fixed period as to how long case histories should be kept, but the Veterinary Defence Society recommends that providing there is no likelihood of litigation, then case details should be kept for a minimum of 2 years. The RCVS suggest longer – 6 years. If however there has been any contention about a case, then the records should be kept for at least 6 years and 364 days.

4. B   **The monitor of a computer can be called a VDU**

VDU stands for Visual Display Unit. The other acronyms also relate to computer terminology:

CPU is Central Processing Unit

CD-ROM is Computer Disk, Read Only Memory

RAM is Random Access Memory – the amount of memory actually on the computer hardware.

5. C   **An active client is one who has visited the practice within a given period of time**

Bonded clients are those that not only have attended the surgery within this time frame, but also have kept vaccinations up to date, and therefore have shown regular attendance at the surgery.

6. C   **Schedule 3 of the Veterinary Surgeons Act 1966 states that a qualified listed veterinary nurse may undertake minor acts of surgery**

7. B   **The Health and Safety at Work Act 1974 can be described as an 'enabling Act'**

This is because it is set out in very broad terms, and it is only by checking the underlying Regulations that the full detail of the law can be determined. It means that if Government wishes to change part of the legislation, only the Regulations pertaining to that particular area need be altered.

It is possible that the Veterinary Surgeons Act may, when updated, become an enabling Act.

8. A   **A minor civil law case is usually heard in the County Court**

More major cases, which might involve large sums in compensation, are more likely to be held in the High Court.

Criminal law cases are tried in either the Magistrates Court, or, if they concern a more serious or indictable offence, the Crown Court.

9. B   **Under current systems of work, the veterinary surgeon is accountable for the actions of a qualified listed veterinary nurse**

At present, if a client made a complaint about the care a nurse gave his/her animal, then the responsibility would rest with the veterinary surgeon, since veterinary nurses do not have any direct professional accountability for their actions. This may change in the future.

10. D   **The Health and Safety at Work Act 1974 provides protection for all people entering a workplace**

The Health and Safety at Work Act sets out basic guidelines for businesses to ensure that all people entering the premises are protected. More specific details about the different types of potential hazards are given in Regulations, such as the Ionising Radiations Regulations 1999.

11. D   The Control of Substances Hazardous to Health Regulations 1999 are not associated with the safe disposal of waste

COSHH Regulations cover the way in which companies should assess and manage the risk associated with the use of chemicals and pharmaceutical products. A business should always aim to use the safest product that is able to fulfil the requirements.

The Control of Pollution Act 1974, the Controlled Waste Regulations 1992 and the Environmental Protection Act 1990 together regulate how businesses should categorise and deal with the different types of waste that are generated.

12. B   Special waste should be placed in rigid yellow plastic tubs, and then collected and incinerated by an authorised company

Special waste includes bottles and vials that had contained pharmaceuticals.

Clinical waste is waste that is contaminated with animal tissues, blood, other body fluids or excretions, and this should be collected and stored in yellow sacks prior to incineration.

Cadavers may be buried by the owners at home, or if they are to be collected from the surgery, must be stored in appropriately coloured sacks, and then incinerated either individually or with other bodies by an authorised company.

Non-clinical commercial waste requires no special treatment.

13. B   If a client was bitten by her cat, this would not normally need to be reported to the HSE under the provisions of RIDDOR

RIDDOR stands for Reporting of Infectious Diseases and Dangerous Occurrences Regulations, and states that if certain types of accidents or illnesses occur at the practice, then the local HSE office should be informed. The type of problems included are:

i. Major or fatal accidents, which include fractures to long bones, amputations of hands or feet, or any other injury that results in someone needing to be detained in hospital for over 24 hours

ii. 'Three day' accidents, which are any accident that causes someone to be absent from work for over 3 days

iii. Certain infectious diseases which include leptospirosis

iv. Dangerous occurrences, such as explosions or uncontrolled release of chemicals or radiation

Therefore it would only be necessary to inform the HSE about the bitten client if she was subsequently unable to work for more than 3 days due to the bite.

14. D   MEL stands for Maximum Exposure Limits

This defines the maximum dose of a substance that any individual may be exposed to. If this exceeded then this should be reported.

15. C   The symbol indicates that the chemical is corrosive

There are separate warning symbols for each of the other hazards.

6 Nutrition

1. C   Dilated cardiomyopathy has been recorded in cats which have been fed taurine-deficient diets

Other problems with a lack of taurine include central retinal degeneration leading to blindness, reproductive problems and impaired immune function.

The other conditions listed can be seen with a number of other nutritional imbalances, but are not totally specific to one nutrient.

2. C   It is true that dietary fats are important in the diet as carriers of fat-soluble vitamins

However, this is not the only reason dietary fat is important. Most dietary fats are made of a glycerol molecule attached to three fatty acid chains, to form triglycerides. Three fatty acids found in fats are described as being essential, and without these some of the fats needed in the body cannot be synthesised.

Fat is also a very valuable energy source – 1 gram of fat provides over twice as many calories as the same quantity of protein or carbohydrate.

3. A   The disease condition unrelated to lack of calcium is hyperthyroidism

Calcium and phosphorus should be present in the diet in approximately equal quantities. If this is not the case, a number of problems may arise. Hyperparathyroidism may result, as high levels of parathyroid hormone (PTH) are released to try and break down bone tissue to release more calcium into the bloodstream. This results in bone weakening and an increased likelihood of fractures. In the growing animal it may also lead to the development of rickets, where long bones do not grow straight. Eclampsia is slightly different, since in this condition the bitch may be receiving what should be adequate amounts of calcium in the diet, but she is simply giving too much away within the milk she is producing for the pups.

4. C   **Lack of potassium in the bloodstream is described as hypokalaemia**

Hyponatraemia refers to a lack of sodium. Hypocupraemia means a lack of copper, and hypocalcaemia is a lack of calcium in the bloodstream.

5. D   **The trace element which has an anti-oxidant function in the body is selenium**

The other trace elements all have quite different roles. Iron is needed for haemoglobin synthesis, iodine is used in the formation of the thyroid hormones and manganese is required in many enzymes, including some involved in carbohydrate and lipid metabolism.

6. B   **The biological value of a protein is a measure of its digestibility and quality**

Proteins with high biological value are very digestible and have a high proportion of essential amino acids in their structure.

7. D   **Vitamin A is also known as retinol**

Many of the vitamins have alternative chemical names which are widely used. Calciferol is vitamin D, thiamine is vitamin B_1 and ascorbic acid is vitamin C.

8. C   **Vitamin K is fat soluble**

There are four fat soluble vitamins:, A, D, E and K. This is an important reason for needing to eat fat in the diet. The other vitamins, the B group vitamins and vitamin C, are water soluble.

9. A   The name given to water generated through chemical reactions within the body is metabolic water

If complex molecules such as amino acids, carbohydrates or fats are broken down to release energy, one of the by-products often produced is water. This contributes to the animal's daily water requirements, and usually meets about 10% of the animal's need.

10. D   The problem with feeding animals raw egg is that it contains avidin, which binds biotin, and reduces its availability

There are a number of foods that contain products that may be detrimental to health if fed in large amounts. Raw fish contains thiaminases, and can lead to vitamin B_1 deficiency. Cereals contain phytates and liver contains high levels of vitamin A. This can cause serious problems due to production of new bone particularly along the spine and around joints. It is a painful condition, and joint movement becomes restricted, making it difficult for the animal to move easily. This is seen particularly in cats, who often develop a taste for raw liver, and become almost addicted to it.

11. A   It is true that cats have only a limited ability to break down carbohydrates, which makes them intolerant of high carbohydrate diets

Cats are obligate carnivores; they are unable to cope with low protein diets and find them very unpalatable. There are also several nutrients they require in the diet that are only found in animal tissues. These include taurine, vitamin A and arachidonic acid. This is quite different from the dog which is an omnivore and is in fact able to survive well on a vegetarian diet if necessary. It is important to appreciate that foods prepared for the two species are quite different, and therefore should not be fed to the other for any length of time.

12. C   When feeding a pregnant bitch it is not necessary to increase food levels until the 5ᵗʰ or 6ᵗʰ week

Increasing food before this will just encourage the bitch to lay down fat, which may actually make parturition more difficult.

Supplements of calcium and Vitamin D are sometimes given in an attempt to prevent the development of eclampsia. However this has been shown not to work if given before it is needed, and might even increase the likelihood of it occurring.

The amount of food that the bitch requires increases steadily from about the 5ᵗʰ week of pregnancy, and continues throughout lactation until the pups start to be weaned. After this there will be a gradual decline in her requirements. The actual amounts do vary with different breeds, and with differing litter size.

13. A   Imbalances in vitamin C levels are not implicated in developmental skeletal abnormalities

Oversupplementation with calcium, or with vitamins A and D (such as by giving cod liver oil) has been proven to lead to skeletal problems. It is far better to feed a proprietary diet that has been formulated for growth. There are even diets specifically for giant breeds designed to ensure that the correct rate of growth is achieved, and muscle development does not outstrip the rate of skeletal maturation.

There is a strange bone condition known as metaphyseal osteopathy (also called hypertrophic osteodystrophy or skeletal scurvy), and this was originally thought to be due to lack of vitamin C. This is now thought not to be the case, but it is not clear what the contributing factors are.

14. B   A kitten should weigh between 600 g and 1000 g by the time it is weaned

15. A   Generally, older cats do not require a reduced calorie intake compared with when they were younger

Basal metabolic rates in cats tend to remain the same

throughout their lives. However, digestive function may decline, so if anything cats may need to be fed more in old age than previously. Dogs, on the other hand, have a lower energy requirement – usually 20% less than before – and so food quantities should be reduced to match this or obesity will be a problem.

To ensure that animals get the nutrients they require it is important that good quality food sources are used and that these are very digestible. Thus protein sources with high biological value should be used.

In disease conditions such as cardiac or renal disease, the restriction of certain minerals may ease the problems these animals might encounter. Therefore it is certainly appropriate to restrict phosphorus intake for renal patients, and sodium for an animals with cardiac conditions.

16. B   The most common presenting sign in animals with dietary sensitivity is pruritus and self-trauma

In cats, this often presents around the head and face, but in dogs it is usually more generalised.

Diarrhoea is seen in some food intolerances such as lactose intolerance or gluten-sensitive enteropathies, but this is specific to these particular problems.

17. B   Exclusion diets should be tried for at least 3 weeks to see if they benefit an animal with suspected dietary sensitivity

For some individuals the signs resolve quite slowly, and it may be necessary to continue on the exclusion diet for longer, for the damaged areas to heal.

18. D   Rapid weight loss in obese cats can lead to the development of hepatic lipidosis

In this condition the liver is infiltrated by fat as a result of the animal's altered metabolism, and this will affect liver function. It is potentially fatal, so programmed weight loss in cats should always be a gradual process.

The other conditions listed in the question are all associated with obesity, so if weight is lost by an obese animal, these diseases should improve.

19. A   It would be useful to provide fats in the form of medium chain triglycerides in cases of malabsorption

Malabsorption problems mean that there is some form of obstruction or prevention of normal absorption of nutrients across the intestinal wall. To support animals with this type of problem, diets should be fed that contain very simple nutrients that are already in a form that can be easily absorbed so that there is maximum opportunity for this to take place as the food passes through the gut. Medium chain triglycerides are relatively easily absorbed and are a valuable source of energy.

Managing the other disease conditions requires other alterations to diet. Colitis and diabetes mellitus are both considered to be fibre responsive diseases, so in many cases increasing fibre in the diet may help. This, however, is not necessarily the case in cats.

Pancreatitis cases should be fed easily digestible, high carbohydrate, low fat diets after an initial period of nil by mouth (usually 2 – 5 days) has been completed.

20. B   It is not possible to actually dissolve calcium oxalate uroliths by dietary modification

The best way to get rid of the uroliths is by surgical removal, and then follow this with a diet that promotes urination, and contains reduced amounts of calcium and oxalate.

The other statements are true about other uroliths – struvite uroliths may be dissolved if the urine is acidified, ammonium urate crystals are seen mostly in Dalmatians, and urates can be prevented from reforming by the use of allopurinol and protein restriction.

21. D   The mineral lost in urine during prolonged use of frusemide diuretic is potassium

Frusemide causes potassium depletion if used for long periods of time, and animals on longterm cardiac management, for example, should therefore be given potassium supplementation. Lack of potassium leads to dysfunction of the excitable cells of the body, which includes nerve and muscle cells.

7 Genetics and animal breeding

1. B   The name given to the chromosomes in the nucleus that are not the X and Y chromosomes is autosomes

The autosomes are found in matched pairs, sometimes referred to as homologous pairs. One chromosome of the pair is inherited from each parent.

The sex chromosomes (X and Y) are also in pairs; the animal is either XX (female) or XY (male).

The term alleles refers to the two different versions of a gene that exist in the cell – one on each of the paired chromosomes.

There is no such term as homosomes.

2. B   The statement that sex-limited genes are only expressed in one sex is true

Sex-limited genes usually code for a characteristic that is only seen in the male or female of a species, despite being present in the genetic makeup of both sexes. Thus a bull may carry genes for good milk quality, or a queen may have the necessary genes for a high sperm count, but they will never be expressed in these individuals.

Sex-linked genes are found on the non-pairing segments of the X and Y chromosomes. They can code for almost any characteristic and are not necessarily related to the sex of the animal.

3. D   The term that describes an animal which has two different alleles for the same gene is heterozygous

If the two alleles were identical, then the animal would be homozygous for that gene. Under normal circumstances, the only time an animal is hemizygous (has just one allele) is in the male animal when it has one X and one Y chromosome. It will therefore only have one copy of most of the genes on these chromosomes.

The term homologous literally means 'same locations', and is used to describe the pairs of chromosomes which have identical gene positions along their lengths.

4. C   **If two heterozygous animals are mated, a quarter of the offspring should show the recessive characteristic**

To show how this works, consider that we are dealing with a gene F, where the dominant allele can be written as a capital F, and the recessive one as a lowercase f.

If the parents are both heterozygous then they must both have the genetic makeup Ff. A table can be drawn to show the possible outcomes of the cross:

	x		Parent 1's alleles	
			F	f
Parent 2's alleles		F	FF	Ff
		f	Ff	ff

Only the young with the genetic makeup ff will show the recessive characteristic, and these make up just a quarter of the possible outcomes.

In reality this does not always appear to work, since if there is a small litter it is less likely to show all the possible genetic outcomes from the cross.

5. B   **The external appearance of an animal is termed its phenotype**

The animal's genetic makeup is its genotype.

Epistasis refers to the situation when one gene masks the expression of another at a different gene locus.

Epistaxis is the word for a nose-bleed.

6. A   **The correct sequence of events during mitosis is prophase, metaphase, anaphase, telophase**

7. C   **An ovum can be referred to as a gamete**

The term gamete is used to describe the sex cells, sperm and ova, which only contain half the genetic information of the normal cells in the body. When the two cells fuse, then the fertilised egg is called a zygote.

Stem cells are cells which are relatively undifferentiated, and can act as a parent cell to a line of cells. Examples include stem cells in the bone marrow able to produce the granulocytes.

Altered genes can result in one of two things happening – either the gene does not work at all, or it works in a different way. This could be beneficial to the animal and result in the development of a new trait, or it could be detrimental, even lethal.

8. D   **The F1 generation is a term used to describe the offspring of animals that are to be mated**

If these offspring are then mated, then their young would be referred to as the F2 generation.

The original animals that are to be mated are the parent generation.

9. A   **The two genes that are most likely to show linkage are the two genes found on the same chromosome**

Two genes on the same chromosome stand a reasonable chance of being inherited together. The closer they are together the more likely this is to happen, and the linkage is described as being close.

Genes on different chromosomes show no linkage since the chance of them being inherited together is random.

Genes on the X and Y chromosomes are never inherited together since each gamete will only receive an X or a Y chromosome.

10. B **Outbreeding is the term used when two animals are mated that are less closely related than if selected at random**

This is used as a technique to introduce new genes into a line, and can result in the offspring showing 'hybrid vigour' or a superiority over their parents.

Inbreeding is when two closely related animals are mated, whereas line breeding describes the mating of animals which are less closely related. In both these situations, the aim is to increase homozygosity of desirable genes. However, the effect may also be to increase the chance of the young being homozygous for undesirable characteristics. This is less likely to occur in line breeding than inbreeding.

11. D **An abnormality or defect present at birth is described as a congenital defect**

The term congenital simply describes when the defect is seen, but gives no explanation as to why it has occurred. Some of these defects are inherited problems, but others could be the result of infection, or exposure to some toxin during the pregnancy.

Phenocopy describes a more unusual situation where a defect is seen that can be inherited, but in this particular animal, was caused by an environmental factor.

12. C **Copper toxicosis has been reported in the Bedlington Terrier as a result of a genetic defect**

There are many breed defects caused by genetic problems, and it is worth being aware of some of the more common problems and the breeds in which these conditions might be seen.

8 Exotic pets and wildlife

1. D   **In rabbits, most breakdown of cellulose and other plant materials takes place in the caecum**

2. C   **Gerbils have a large skin gland on the mid-ventral abdomen**

This occasionally gets infected, and animals may present at the surgery with swelling in this area.

Rabbits are the species that do not have any pads on the feet, and the females have a dewlap – the fold of skin under the chin.

Hamsters have glandular areas on their flanks, and the skin is often darkly pigmented in this area.

3. D   **Canaries are members of the order Passeriformes**

The Passeriformes include perching birds such as the canary and members of the finch family.

The Psittaciformes include the parrots, the Anseriformes include ducks, geese and swans, and the Galliformes include poultry, pheasants and quail.

4. B   **Birds have two digits in the wing**

Digit III still remains at the wingtip, and the alula or bastard wing is formed from digit I. The feathers on the alula are important for control at take off and landing.

5. B   **The crop is the organ in which food is stored prior to digestion**

The crop is found part way down the neck, and it is simply a pocket formed ventrally from the oesophagus. Not all birds have a crop – owls and diving birds often do not.

Food moves on from the oesophagus into the proventriculus, the equivalent of the mammalian stomach, where enzyme digestion is started. After this organ lies the gizzard or ventriculus, which is where the food is ground. Species that require grit use it in the gizzard to increase the grinding effect.

In herbivorous or omnivorous species there are often two large caeca, which is where most bacterial breakdown of plant material takes place.

6. D   Gaseous exchange takes place within the lungs of birds

Although the way in which the respiratory system works in birds is quite different to other species, it is important to realise that the areas where oxygen and carbon dioxide are exchanged is still the lungs.

Air is drawn through the lungs into air sacs as the bird breathes in. Gas is exchanged during this movement, and then again when the bird exhales. The air sacs are found throughout the body and may even extend into some bones, but these are thin-walled structures and are not involved in gas exchange.

7. C   Ectothermic animals may aestivate when temperatures are too high

When this happens the animals become lethargic and tend to sleep. High temperatures will cause animals to do this, but so will very dry conditions; many reptiles have a requirement for minimum levels of humidity.

8. A   Snakes have only one functional lung

Snakes and lizards have certain anatomical differences from mammals which relate to their elongated shape. In both species the lungs are quite elongated, but in the snake only one is functional.

9. A   The term ovo-viviparous describes animals which retain their eggs within their bodies until the young are ready to hatch

Viviparous species give birth to live young which have been nurtured via a placenta, as is the case for mammals.

Oviparous animals lay eggs which then require incubation before the young are ready to hatch.

Finally, the only species in which the male holds the young in his abdomen is the seahorse. There are not many fathers like this around!

10. D   An adult guinea pig requires 50 mg vitamin C per day

11. A   Rabbits are induced ovulators

All the other species listed are spontaneous ovulators. This means that they will ovulate whether or not they are mated. However, induced ovulators must be mated in order to ovulate.

Rabbits are not the only species that are induced ovulators – ferrets and cats also fit into this category.

12. D   Parrots can live for 40-50 years – or even more!

13. C   Birds of prey being treated by a veterinary surgeon are exempt from the Wildlife and Countryside Act for 6 weeks

If birds are being kept in captivity for longer, they must be ringed and registered.

14. C   Healthy tortoises should not lose up to 3% of their bodyweight per month during hibernation

It is normal for tortoises to lose up to 1% per month, but losses above this are abnormal, and the animal should be brought out of hibernation if this occurs.

15. A   The term that describes the shedding of skin, as snakes do, is ecdysis

Autotomy is the shedding of the tail. This can happen in lizards if they are picked up by the tail.

Setae are the irritating hairs found on the limbs of the tarantula. These can cause skin reactions in people, so gloves should be worn when handling these species.

Myiasis is the correct term for fly-strike, commonly seen in rabbits, but also possible in any other species on which the blue and green bottle flies lay their eggs.

16. D   Plants should be soaked in a solution of potassium permanganate before setting up an aquarium

The plants should be soaked in a solution of 2 parts per million of potassium permanganate for 48 hours, and then placed in the aquarium. New aquaria should then be allowed to settle for 2 weeks before any fish are added.

17. B   Guinea pigs may show 'barbering'

Guinea pigs may barber or chew each other's fur if there is insufficient fibre in the diet. This seems to be specific to guinea pigs, and is not reported in the other breeds listed.

18. D   Psittacosis is a disease seen in birds that can also cause problems in humans

Chlamydia psittaci is an organism that is zoonotic and can cause, flu-like symptoms in people. PBFD is a viral disease that affects the bird's skin, and birds will often pluck their own feathers. It is very contagious, and not easy to treat, being a virus. However, it is not zoonotic.

Trichomoniasis is caused by a protozoan that affects the oesophagus and crop, leading to regurgitation and depressed appetite.

Newcastle disease is another viral disease.

19. A   A blood sample from a tortoise should be collected from the jugular vein

The cephalic vein is often used for venous access in cats and dogs, and can also be used in the larger exotic mammals such as ferrets and rabbits. However it is more common to use the marginal ear vein in rabbits.

The ventral tail vein provides venous access for a number of species including snakes, lizards and the small mammals such as mice (providing suitable restraint can be provided).

20. A   Jackson's ratio provides a useful indicator of health in the tortoise

In order to determine whether a tortoise is the correct weight or not, measurements should be taken of the length of the plastron and the tortoise then weighed. The figures should then be compared with a graph showing the average weight:length ratio. From this it can be determined how close the tortoise is to the ideal ratio. This can be particularly important prior to hibernation, since underweight tortoises may not survive, and it may be preferable to keep the tortoise awake over the winter months.

Similar judgements can be made for birds. These use a comparison between weight and the length of the ulna.

21. D   Both snakes and tortoises require fasting prior to anaesthesia

Snakes can vomit, so like cats and dogs should be starved before an anaesthetic. Chelonians do not usually vomit, but they too require starving or there may be significant compression of the lungs during anaesthesia.

9 Medicines: pharmacology, therapeutics and dispensing

1. A   **The therapeutic index of a drug is the ratio between the dose that causes toxic effects and the dose that provides the desired effect**

The pharmacodynamics of a drug define the type of action that the drug has in the body, and its pharmoacokinetics describe how it is absorbed, metabolised and excreted by the body.

The dose of a drug that experimentally causes death in 50% of the animals tested is referred to as the LD50 for that product, and is a measure of its toxicity.

2. D   **Bacteriostatic drugs prevent the multiplication of bacteria**

Bacteriostatic drugs are used to control the numbers of bacteria within the body. The actual killing and removal of the bacteria is then carried out by the animal's immune system.

Bactericidal products kill bacteria.

At present there are no drugs which can be used against all micro-organisms without also causing harm to the host species.

3. B   **Acyclovir is used as an antiviral product**

Nystatin is an antifungal agent. Fenbendazole is an anthelminthic (particularly good against roundworms) and amoxycillin is a penicillin-based antibiotic.

4. C   The drug used in cardiac disease that acts on the heart to increase the force of cardiac contraction is pimobendan (Vetmedin)

Drugs with this effect can be referred to as positive inotropes.

Lignocaine is sometimes used to suppress cardiac dysrhythmias. Enalapril (Enacard) causes peripheral venous and arterial dilation, and therefore reduces the resistance to blood flow, making it easier for the heart to push the blood round the body.

Propanolol is commonly referred to as a β-blocker. Drugs of this type slow down the heart rate (negative chronotropes).

5. C   Barbiturates can be used in the treatment or management of epilepsy

Antimuscarinic drugs have a number of different names including anticholinergics (acting against nerve cells containing acetyl choline i.e. parasympathetic neurons) and antisialogogues (preventing salivation). These reduce salivation and bronchial secretions, and increase heart rate. They may be included in a premedicant regime.

Muscle relaxants are ONLY used whilst animals are under general anaesthesia, and these cause relaxation of all the skeletal muscles, including the respiratory muscles. Patients must therefore be ventilated.

Local anaesthetics are generally used to provide local analgesia by preventing nerve impulses in nearby neurons.

6. D   Carprofen (Zenecarp) is the non-steroidal anti-inflammatory drug licensed for use as part of a premedication in small animals

The only other product licensed for this purpose in small animals is Meloxicam (Metacam). Other products have not been given licenses since they are not as specific for the inflammatory prostaglandins as the two products detailed above.

7. B **Astringents are used on skin to leave a protective coating of protein**

Products such as calamine lotion would come into this category of drugs. Keratolytics are very different – they are used on skin, but act to loosen the keratinised squames on the surface of the skin so that they separate from the epidermis beneath.

Mucolytics work in the respiratory tract and eyes, and prevent or reduce mucus production. Mydriatics also affect the eyes and cause pupil dilation or mydriasis.

8. B **Toxoids do not contain preformed antibodies to toxin**

Toxoids actually contain quantities of a toxin which has been altered so that it does not cause harm to the animal. However it is still close enough to the original to stimulate production of appropriate antibodies which will protect the animal in the future. It is the same for a vaccine; the only difference is that a vaccine contains altered or killed organism rather than toxin.

Antisera and antitoxins both play the same role. These contain preformed antibodies that can be given to an animal in the face of a disease to provide some instant protection. These do not last long in the circulation, but hopefully long enough to get an animal through an acute crisis. The only difference between them is that antisera contain antibodies to organisms, and antitoxins contain antibodies to toxins.

9. B **The concentration of a 1.25% solution in mg/ml is 12.5 mg/ml**

In order to work this out, you need to be aware of the definition of a percentage solution.

A 1% solution, by definition, contains 1 g of drug in 100 ml

Therefore, a 1.25% solution must contain 1.25 g of drug in 100 ml.

However, the answer required is in mg/ml, not grams, so it is best to convert the g into mg.

Remember there are 1000 mg in 1 g.

So, 1.25 g is the same as 1.25 x 1000 mg = 1250 mg.

Which means that the solution contains 1250 mg in 100 ml.

For the final step we need to work out how many mg are in 1 ml.

To do, this all that is required is to divide the quantity in 100 ml by 100.

Therefore the concentration in mg/ml = 1250 ÷ 100
                                                            = 12.5 mg/ml.

N.B. If you find the maths hard, there is another way to do these – simply remember that to convert from % to mg/ml, all you need to do is to multiply by 10. It will always work!

10. A   The product that should be used as a last resort is one which has no product license for animal or human use

Under the cascade, drugs should be prescribed in the following order, and drugs from lower levels should not be used if drugs from the levels above exist.

i.   A drug that is licensed in the particular species for the condition to be treated

ii. A drug licensed for use in another species for the same condition or in the same species but for a different condition

iii. A drug with a human product license

iv. A drug with no product license

11. D   Only General Sales List products may be sold to someone at a surgery without the vet having seen their animal

All other classes of drugs can only be dispensed to owners whose animals are under the veterinary surgeon's care, and have been seen in the recent past. The precise timing of 'recent past' often depends on the nature of the product – a year may be quite appropriate for flea treatments, whereas a vet may not wish to dispense cardiac drugs without having seen the animal within the last three months, since cardiac disease may change quite rapidly.

12. C Products for external use should be dispensed in coloured fluted bottles, if not in the manufacturer's original packaging

Plain bottles should be reserved for internal medications. This is to enable quick distinction between internal and external products by someone partially sighted or even blind.

Loose tablets or capsules should be dispensed in plastic or glass pots, preferably with child-proof lids. However, elderly clients may find these difficult, so it is also worth keeping a few screw-top pots too. Only pre-packaged medicines (e.g. sachets or tablets/capsules in blister packs) may be dispensed in paper or cardboard envelopes.

Wide-mouthed jars are probably best for powders or creams.

13. C Legally, it is not essential to include the quantity and strength of drug on the label of a dispensed product

However, it is considered poor practice if this is not done! All the other information is essential.

14. D The Misuse of Drugs Act 1971 gives details about the use, storage and supply of Controlled Drugs

This has been added to by the Misuse of Drugs Regulations introduced in 1985 and updated in 2001.

The Medicines Act 1968 describes the basic classification of products into POM, P, PML and GSL, and gives information about storage, use and supply of all medicines.

The Health and Safety at Work Act and the COSHH Regulations are broad pieces of legislation that cover many aspects of safety in the workplace and the use of all chemicals, not just pharmaceutical products.

15. D Diazepam is a Schedule 4 drug

Schedule 4 contains products of relatively low abuse potential, such as some of the tranquillisers. It also includes some anabolic steroids.

Schedule 1 products are the most addictive, and have no

current medical use in the UK. Cannabis is in this class, but there may be changes to make this a Schedule 2 product since there have been good reports of its benefit to human patients with multiple sclerosis. However, there are no veterinary indications for its use.

Schedule 2 products are still potentially addictive, but have medical value – so this includes morphine and other opium derivatives.

Schedule 3 products include the barbiturates, and a couple of opiates which are less prone to abuse.

Schedule 5 products are those which contain very small amounts of controlled drugs, such as kaolin and morphine mixtures used for the treatment of diarrhoea.

16. B   A Controlled Drugs register should be kept for 2 years after the last entry

This allows Customs and Excise to trace all usage of the controlled drugs. Any drugs that are out of date should be disposed of in the presence of a Home Office Inspector who is required to sign the entry in the Register.

17. C   The abbreviation used on a prescription that means 'every 8 hours' is q8h

om means every morning.

prn means as required.

tbs is the abbreviation for a tablespoon.

10 Laboratory diagnostic aids

1. C   A Pasteur pipette would be suitable to decant off plasma from a centrifuged blood sample

This does not require precise measurement of the volume involved, and a dropping pipette such as the Pasteur is fine. All the others are used to measure accurate volumes of fluid.

2. A   The part of the microscope that holds the objective lenses is the nosepiece

The nosepiece is a rotating turret into which several objective lenses can be screwed. The appropriate lens can then be rotated into position over the slide.

The mechanical stage is the platform on which the slide rests. It is described as mechanical if the position of the slide can be moved by control knobs at the side of the stage, rather than simply by pushing the slide with fingers.

The condenser is a lens found underneath the stage. Its function is to focus light from the light source onto the object on the slide to give maximum definition.

The body of the microscope is the part of the microscope lying between the objective lens and the eye pieces.

3. D   The x40 objective can be referred to as the high dry lens

This is the highest power lens usually found on a microscope that is to be used dry – i.e. without oil.

4. C   Bacteria are usually cultured at a temperature of 37°C

5. B   EDTA is the best anticoagulant for haematological studies

Heparin is used for most biochemical analyses, with the exception of blood glucose estimations for which fluoride oxalate should be used. Sodium citrate is used for coagulation studies and erythrocyte sedimentation studies (rarely carried out in practice nowadays).

6. C   Cystocentesis is the best method of urine collection if the sample is to be cultured for bacteria

Cystocentesis is the only method of urine collection in which there is no external contamination of the sample. Catheterisation also gives a representative sample, but there may be additional cells from the urethra displaced by the catheter into the sample, and there is the risk of urethral trauma.

Mid-stream samples and those obtained by manual expression are the least useful, since external contaminants from the coat or the environment can end up within the sample. The urine may also be contaminated by cells from the genital system.

7. B   The pot should not be filled to a maximum of a quarter full

Pots in which faeces samples are collected should be filled as full as possible. This means that there is minimum exposure to air of the sample, since this could affect the bacteria and parasites that might be present.

Fresh samples should certainly be used, and if this means rectal samples are required, then make sure the animal is well restrained, your nails are short and gloves are worn.

Faeces should be examined as soon as possible since some of the parasites and bacteria deteriorate very quickly, so far greater accuracy will be achieved if analysis is carried out within an hour of collection.

Collection of faeces per rectum may also stimulate the animal to urinate. Therefore, if urine samples are needed too, then it is best to collect these first to avoid missing the moment!

8. D   Hair plucks are most suitable for the diagnosis of ringworm

Yeasts such as malassezia can be collected using tape techniques or skin swabs.

Surface-dwelling mites, such as cheyletiella, can be collected very easily using tape, but burrowing mites like sarcoptes are more difficult to find and usually require several fairly deep skin scrapes.

Bacterial infections can be identified by taking swabs or occasionally using tape preparations.

9. C   The largest fluid sample that can be sent through the post is 50 ml

Samples sent through the post must conform to postal regulations, and this includes a maximum volume of 50 ml. The sample must be securely sealed, and then surrounded in sufficient absorbent material to absorb all the fluid should the primary container leak.

If you send samples via couriers to external laboratories, you may find that their requirements are different. Always check with the laboratory before sending a sample.

10. A   Brilliant cresyl blue is an example of a supra-vital stain

Supra-vital staining techniques are used to stain reticulocytes. The blood is actually cultured with the stain, and cells take up the stain. Organelles show up as dark blue strands, and even though the organelles in reticulocytes are gradually being ejected from the cell, remnants can still be seen when samples are made into smears and examined under the microscope.

The other stains listed are all Romanowsky stains which contain a mix of methylene blue and eosin, so that acidic areas stain red, and basic areas stain blue.

11. B   A normal white cell count in the dog is 6-18 x 10^9/l

Normal red cell count in the dog is 5.5-8.5 x 10^{12}/l

Notice the difference in the power – there are about 1000 times more red cells than white cells, so the power difference is 3 – the same as the number of zeros in 1000.

12. C   Howell-Jolly bodies are found in reticulocytes

These are the remnants of the nucleus of the red cell which are seen in reticulocytes before they develop into mature erythrocytes.

13. A   Lymphocytes are usually seen in increased numbers with viral conditions

Lymphocytes have two roles in the body – to produce antibodies and to provide cell-mediated immunity. These are both very important in the fight against viral infections, so the number of these types of cells often increases in these infections.

Monocytes are involved in the removal of cell debris, and monocytosis is quite unusual. An eosinophilia may be seen in allergic conditions or heavy parasitism.

Neutrophils are particularly involved in fighting bacteria and so numbers increase in the body if there is a bacterial infection.

14. C   ALT is more specific in small animals than AST

ALT is an enzyme found solely in liver cells in small animals, and so raised levels indicate that there is ongoing liver damage. AST is found not just in liver cells, but also in skeletal and cardiac muscle cells. Therefore damage to any of these tissues will result in a rise in AST levels.

BUN and urea levels are not identical and do not have the same value. The BUN is lower, since this is a measure of the quantity of just the nitrogen contained within the urea, rather than the whole urea molecule.

Glucose levels vary considerably throughout the day. Factors that cause variation include whether the animal has exercised or just eaten, so if blood samples are to be analysed for glucose, then a fasting sample should be taken, and it is usual that samples are taken first thing in the morning having starved the animal overnight.

Creatinine is a by-product of protein metabolism, and is normally excreted by the kidney. However it has no relation to the liver, and therefore no reflection on its function. This is different from urea, since ammonia and amines are converted to urea by the liver before excretion by the kidney.

15. D **Potassium hydroxide clears the slide of cellular debris, and makes it easier to examine hair shafts for evidence of ringworm, or ectoparasites**

Potassium hydroxide can help clear slides, particularly if the sample is heated before examination by passing it through a Bunsen flame. It has no staining properties.

16. A **Sudan III can be used to show up undigested fat in a faecal smear**

Sudan III will stain any fat globules a bright orange colour.

Lugol's iodine can be used to check for undigested starch which shows up as blue-black granules within the smear.

Eosin, Sudan III and new methylene blue can all be used to check for undigested muscle fibres. The dyes help to show up the striations and the nuclei of the cells.

17. B **Urine samples should be centrifuged at 1,500 rpm for 5 minutes in order to separate sediment from supernatant**

1,500 rpm is often used as an appropriate speed for centrifugation if the material that sinks is still to be examined. This is therefore true in faecal sedimentation techniques as well as urine analysis.

If the cells are not to be examined, and the reason for centrifuging is simply to determine how much space they occupy (as for PCV readings) then the speed can be considerably faster. 10,000 rpm is usually used for PCV measurements.

18. A **An animal needs to be kept on a meat-free diet for 3 days before its faeces can be tested for occult blood**

If animals are not kept off meat, the tests that detect hidden or occult blood will give false positives, since myoglobin cross-reacts with haemoglobin.

19. C **The original reading for the urine sample was 1.064**

In order to work out an original SG, simply ignore the first digit, 1. Then depending on the dilution used, the later figure should be multiplied. In this case the dilution was 1 part urine to 1 part water (2 parts total) so the .032 should be multiplied by 2.

If the dilution had been 1 part urine to 2 parts water (3 parts total), then the multiplication factor would have been 3, and so on.

Finally, don't forget to replace the first digit 1 at the start of the number you have calculated!

20. B   Ascorbic acid can cause false negatives for glucose if present in urine samples being tested by urine dipsticks

Ascorbic acid can be produced naturally in the intestine of the dog, and so there are occasions in which suppression of the glucose results can occur.

Conversely, dipsticks exposed to hypochlorites (bleach) will lead to false positives.

Blood may cause problems simply by causing discolouration of the patches on the dipsticks.

Bilirubin should not affect the glucose patch on a dipstick.

21. A   Cystine crystals are usually seen as flat hexagons within urine

Calcium oxalate crystals are usually octahedral in shape, and appear as square crystals with a cross through the diagonals (an envelope shape).

Ammonium urate crystals appear like thorn-apples, and struvite crystals are described as looking like coffin lids.

22. D   Methylene blue can be used as a basic stain to determine the presence of bacteria

Leishman's stain is a Romanowsky stain, and is usually used for blood smears.

Lugol's iodine and eosin are both used individually in the examination of faeces. Direct faecal smears can be made, and then stained to check for evidence of maldigestion. Iodine is used to show up undigested starch, and eosin helps identify undigested muscle fibres.

23. D   **Carbol fuschin is used as the counterstain in Gram's stain**

The primary stain is crystal violet, and all bacteria would stain with this stain if it was the only one used. The mordant, Lugol's iodine, fixes the primary stain into the cell wall of Gram-positive bacteria.

Acetone is a decolourant, and when the slide is rinsed with acetone, unfixed primary stain is rinsed off the bacteria. If the slide was examined at this stage, Gram-positive bacteria would be visible as purple cells, but Gram-negative bacteria would not be seen. Therefore a counterstain is used to show these up. Either carbol fuschin or safranin can be used to make these bacteria stain pink so that they can be examined.

24. D   **Urine to be tested for bacteriological growth should be preserved with boric acid**

Thymol and hydrochloric acid can be used if biochemical analysis is to be carried out.

Acetic acid is used if ascorbic acid levels are required.

However, it is preferable to test the sample as soon as possible rather than rely on the use of preservatives. If there is to be a slight delay before testing, urine samples without preservatives can be refrigerated for up to 6 hours without compromising the results.

11 Elementary microbiology and immunology

1. B   **The true statement is that commensal organisms cause no harm or benefit to the host**

However, this situation may change if the host's immune system is compromised, in which case they may cause harm and become opportunist pathogens.

Most micro-organisms are parasitic, and as seen already by the fact that some are commensals, not all are pathogenic. In fact, some help the host – for example, many bacteria found within the intestines of mammals are beneficial, and these are described as mutualistic or symbiotic.

It is certainly not the case that all bacteria secrete toxins, though quite a number do.

Finally, there is an important difference between infectious and contagious. Infectious diseases are simply caused by micro-organisms. Both kennel cough and an abscess are examples, and whilst kennel cough is certainly contagious, it is not really possible to 'catch' an abscess!

2. A   **Endotoxins are produced by Gram-negative bacteria**

Gram-negative bacteria have a slightly different call wall structure to the Gram-positive bacteria, and the extra layer of lipo-polysaccharide (LPS) acts as endotoxin when the cell dies and breaks down. It is therefore different from an exotoxin which is actively secreted by a live bacterium. Exotoxins are only produced by Gram-positive bacteria.

A few fungi secrete toxins – in particular, the fungus Aspergillus can produce a toxin called aflatoxin.

Viruses do not secrete toxins – they usually cause damage

to host cells when the newly-formed virus particles break out of an infected cell, and then invade other cells nearby. Once the virus has replicated, these cells too are damaged.

3. D A disease normally present within an area can be described as endemic

If there is an increase in the level of a particular disease, then it can be described as an epidemic. To be totally accurate, if animal diseases are being referred to then the term epizootic should be used in this situation.

Pandemics are global increases in disease, and this usually happens because a new strain or even a new organism has developed to which the hosts have no previous experience and therefore no immunity.

4. A A toxoid is used to stimulate the development of an animal's immunity against a toxin

Toxoids contain toxins from bacteria that have been altered so that they no longer cause disease, but still stimulate an immune response that would also be effective against the native toxin.

Vaccines are similar, except that they contain actual organism which is either dead, attenuated or in the case of organisms such as feline leukaemia virus, just part of the original organism.

Antiserum and antitoxin both contain pre-made antibodies; the former against organisms, the latter against toxins. These are used to provide instant protection in the face of disease. The antibodies are not long lasting, so the use of these would not replace a vaccination programme.

5. B Bacteria with a curved rod shape can be classed as vibrios

Campylobacter is an example of a vibrio.

Bacilli are straight rods and examples include E. coli and Salmonella.

Cocci are round bacteria, and Staphylococcus and Streptococcus are both examples of this type.

Spirochaetes are spiral-shaped bacteria, and examples include Leptospira and Borrelia species.

6. D   A facultative anaerobe grows best in the presence of oxygen, but will grow in its absence

Different bacteria have different growth preferences. Some bacteria can only grow in the presence of oxygen – obligate aerobes – others can only grow in the absence of oxygen – obligate anaerobes.

Some. however, have the capability to cope if conditions are not quite perfect, and as mentioned above facultative anaerobes would come into this section. Facultative aerobes are the opposite – bacteria that grow best without oxygen, but if it is present are still able to multiply.

Microaerophiles are those that grow best in small quantities of oxygen.

7. C   Bacteria from the genus Clostridium are able to produce spores

All the spore-forming bacteria are Gram-positive organisms, and most of them are either in the genus Clostridium (such as Clostridium tetani which causes tetanus) or Bacillus (such as Bacillus anthracis which causes anthrax).

Streptococcus might be a Gram-positive bacterium, but it is not a spore-forming one, and Escherichia and Salmonella are both Gram-negative and so do not use this survival technique.

8. C   Conjugation is a means by which genetic information may be transferred from one bacterium to another

Conjugation results in the transfer of a plasmid, a small circular piece of DNA, from a donor bacterium to a recipient bacterium. This only seems to occur in Gram-negative species. It is not a form of reproduction, although it is occasionally referred to as 'bacterial mating', since there are no more bacteria after the transfer than before.

Fusion of bacteria does not occur.

9. A   **The medium that encourages the growth of Salmonella whilst inhibiting other bacteria is deoxycholate citrate agar**

MacConkey agar is a nutrient agar with a few modifications. Firstly it contains bile salts. Many bacteria cannot grow in their presence, but most enteric bacteria can. Secondly it contains the carbohydrate lactose and pH indicator dye. If the bacteria ferment and use the lactose, then the colonies become more acidic and show up as pink. Colonies that do not use the lactose, but use other nutrients to grow, remain white.

Blood agar and chocolate agar are very similar and both can be described as enriched media. Blood agar, as its name suggests, has had blood added to the mix, and is useful for growing fastidious organisms that require more than a basic nutrient source. It is also useful to show up bacteria capable of producing haemolysis, since often these are more pathogenic. For example, some strains of Streptococcus are described as being β-haemolytic and these are the type of organisms involved in the disease strangles in horses.

Chocolate agar has got nothing to do with chocolate! This is basically a blood agar except that the mix has been heat treated so that the blood is lysed, and the nutrients within the red cells are even more available. The name comes from the deep chocolate colour of the agar.

10. C   **It is true that viruses always contain nucleic acid and a protein coat**

This is all that is required in the simplest viral structures. The nucleic acid can be DNA or RNA, but never both. The shape of viruses also varies in complexity with many of the simpler viruses being icosahedral, but as well as helical viruses, there are also more complex shapes such as that shown by bacteriophages.

Some viruses cover the outside of the capsid (the protein coat) with an envelope, and this may be formed from the cell membrane of the host cell in which it multiplied. This can be a very effective way for the virus to hide from the host's immune system, since it is now not as obviously 'foreign'. Several viruses do this, and there is no requirement for the virus to have a particular shape – helical or otherwise.

11. A   The type of organism thought to be the cause of Feline Spongiform Encephalopathy is a prion

Prions are small filaments of protein that infect the central nervous system, and eventually cause fatal damage. These have been known about in sheep for some while, but it is more recently that cattle, cats and humans have been diagnosed with this type of particle.

12. D   Interferon is an example of non-specific immunity

If a cell is infected by any virus, then the cell will release a chemical messenger called interferon. This causes neighbouring cells to alter their cell membranes slightly to make it more difficult for viruses to invade. It is non-specific since it is unrelated to the type of virus involved.

There are two types of specific immunity – humoral immunity, the production of specific antibodies by B-lymphocytes, and cell-mediated immunity, in which the T-cells play a number of roles. Some T-cells secrete lymphokines which stimulate other immune cells to act against the infection; some are described as helper cells and these stimulate the appropriate B-cell to produce more antibodies, and some are killer cells, which kill host cells that have been infected by the virus in order to prevent its replication.

In both humoral and cell-mediated immunity it is only the lymphocytes that recognise each particular pathogen that are stimulated to become active.

12 Elementary mycology and parasitology

1. D **The fungus responsible for cases of ringworm in small animals is Trichophyton mentagrophytes**

This is one of two moulds commonly diagnosed as causing ringworm in cats and dogs. The other species is Microsporum canis.

Candida albicans occasionally causes infections on mucous membranes, and is colloquially referred to as 'thrush'.

Aspergillus occasionally causes nasal infections in dogs (aspergillosis), and Malassezia can cause dermatitis and otitis in affected animals.

2. B **Sabouraud's medium should be used for culturing fungi**

The other media listed are all bacterial growth media.

3. B **It is only the larval form of Trombicula autumnalis that is parasitic**

Felicola and Sarcoptes are permanent parasites, and spend all of their life on the host, so all stages of the life cycle are parasitic.

Ctenocephalides is parasitic as an adult, but not during the larval stage, when it lives off organic debris in the environment.

4. B **The sucking louse of the dog is Linognathus setosus**

All the other lice listed are biting lice. Felicola affects cats, Trichodectes affects dogs, and Damalinia infests cattle.

Biting lice and sucking lice can usually be distinguished by the shape of their heads. Biting lice have broad heads, whereas the heads of sucking lice are generally more pointed. Biting lice chew through the external epidermis and cause considerable irritation, whereas the sucking lice suck blood, and may, in large numbers, cause anaemia.

5. D   Pediculosis describes infestation with lice

Of the parasites listed, the only other infestation with a specific name is myiasis, which is infestation with blow fly (dipteran) larvae.

6. B   It is untrue that fleas may carry Taenia hydatigena

Fleas are the intermediate host for Dipylidium caninum, not Taenia species. Taenia usually use mammals as their intermediate hosts.

All the other statements are true.

7. A   Ctenocephalides canis is an insect

Parasitic insects include the fleas, the lice and the larvae of blow flies. All adult insects have six legs and three distinct body parts – head, thorax and abdomen. They are also usually macroscopic.

Sarcoptes and Demodex are both mites, and are therefore arachnids – members of the spider family. Like spiders, the adults have eight legs, and usually only two body sections, the cephalothorax and the abdomen.

Trichophyton is one of the organisms that causes ringworm, and is therefore a fungus.

8. D   Ctenocephalides felis is not host specific

Despite being called the cat flea, this is a very successful parasite due to its ability to utilise many different hosts. So far, C. felis has been found on over 50 different species of host!

All the other parasites listed are quite host specific, and therefore infestations are easier to contain and treat, and pose less zoonotic risk.

9. B   Cnemidocoptes is the burrowing mite that causes scaly leg and scaly beak in cage birds

All the mites listed are burrowing mites, so all can produce obvious hair or fur loss, and most produce intense irritation. Demodex is the only species that does not always cause pruritus.

Notoedres is seen very rarely in cats. Demodex is found in many species, but each host has its own particular subspecies of the mite.

Trixacarus is found in guinea pigs.

10. C   'Walking dandruff' is the nickname given to cheyletiella

Cheyletiella species generally induce very heavy scurf production by the host, due to the irritation that these mites produce. There are several species of Cheyletiella infesting different hosts. Cheyletiella yasguri affects dogs, Cheyletiella parasitovorax affects rabbits and Cheyletiella blakei affects cats.

11. B   It is the larval stage of the life cycle that only has three pairs of legs

The stages in the life cycle of an arachnid are:

Egg – Larva (3 pairs of legs) – Nymph (4 pairs of legs) – Adult (4 pairs of legs)

Arachnids do not pupate, so there is no pupa stage.

It is worth noting how the number of legs changes, since despite being arachnids, parasitic Trombicula larvae will only have 6 legs in total. The same is also true of larval ticks which are often tiny, and could be confused with other parasites.

12. D   An individual segment of a tapeworm is a proglottid

Strobila is the name given to the whole chain of segments that forms behind the head or scolex of the worm. The rostral part of the head is called the rostellum, and there is often a ring of hooks around the rostellum to aid attachment of the tapeworm to the intestinal lining.

13. C   **Echinococcus granulosus forms a hydatid cyst as its intermediate stage**

Hydatid cysts are usually seen in sheep, but occasionally occur in humans if eggs are accidentally ingested. These cysts can grow up to 20 cm in diameter, and may cause problems, depending on the cyst's location.

Other intermediate stages are far smaller. Taenia species form a cysticercus within the intermediate host. These cysts grow up to about 8 cm in diameter.

Dipylidium caninum uses invertebrates as its intermediate host, and the intermediate stage, the cysticercoid, is tiny – it has to be to fit into the abdominal cavity of a flea or a louse!

14. B   **The drug that is effective against all tapeworms is praziquantel**

Some tapeworms are susceptible to fenbendazole and mebendazole, but none can be treated with piperazine. These three products, however, are suitable for treating roundworms, whereas praziquantel is not.

15. A   **It is not true that the larvae of Toxocara canis infest pups by just two routes**

The routes described are quite correct, but it is important to appreciate that pups are infested even before they are born since the larvae are also able to cross the placenta. This is different from Toxocara cati whose life cycle is very similar with the exception that placental transfer does not occur.

Paratenic hosts are perhaps less important in the transfer of Toxocara canis than the other ways in which this worm is spread, but transfer by this route can and does occur.

Another important factor to consider when wishing to control spread of worms is that freshly passed faeces do not pose a hazard, since any worm eggs in the faeces will not yet be infective. The larvae develop within the egg, and it is the second stage larva or L_2 that is the infective form. This takes time to develop, and if faeces are cleared as soon as they are passed, and then incinerated, the eggs will be destroyed before they reach the infective stage.

Visceral larval migrans can, in rare instances, be very serious and cases of partial or complete blindness have been reported where the larva affects the retina of the eye. However, many cases go undetected since the organ in which the larva comes to rest does not lead to the development of clinical signs.

16. D About 10% of adult dogs have a patent infestation of Toxocara canis

In most adult dogs Toxocara canis larvae are dormant within the tissues. However, in about 10% of cases there is a patent infestation, meaning that there are adult worms in the intestine which are shedding eggs into the faeces.

This may be due to stressors affecting the dog, for example pregnancy which causes dormant larvae to be reactivated, or due to the ingestion of paratenic hosts containing the larvae. Therefore regular worming is still recommended in adult animals as well as juveniles.

17. C The eggs of the two worms can be distinguished because Toxocara canis has a rough, pitted shell

The egg of Toxascaris, however, is smooth. The two eggs are quite similar in size, and although colour differences are sometimes mentioned in texts, this may be difficult to appreciate in a faecal sample.

The worm with the lemon-shaped egg is Trichuris vulpis, and the worms which are found as free larvae in the faeces are the lungworms including Oslerus osleri (Filaroides osleri).

18. C Uncinaria stenocephala is the hookworm more commonly seen in dogs in the UK

Both Uncinaria and Ancylostoma are hookworms, but Ancylostoma is more often seen abroad than in the UK.

Trichuris vulpis is the whipworm, and Toxascaris is similar to Toxocara in appearance, though its life cycle is quite different.

19. A   The proper name of the heartworm is Dirofilaria immitis

Dirofilaria is not a common infestation in animals in the UK, and under import schemes animals from areas where the disease is endemic animals are required to be treated prior to entry.

Aelurostrongylus abstrusus is the lungworm of the cat.

Capillaria plica is quite rare in the UK, and lives in the bladder.

Toxoplasma gondii is not a worm at all, but a protozoan.

20. B   Toxoplasma gondii is the parasite that could induce abortion if a woman was infested for the first time during pregnancy

Fortunately this is rare. However it is important that cat owners realise that there is a risk, however small. Toxoplasma infects people in one of two ways – either by contamination of food/water by cat faeces which contain the oocysts, or by ingestion of meat containing schizont cysts containing the intermediate stage of the organism.

It is probably the latter that is the greater risk, since serological studies in the States have shown that people living or working with cats show no greater exposure to the organism than those who have no direct contact with cats. Therefore, whilst pregnant women should avoid handling cat litter trays and wear gloves when gardening, they should also make sure that all meat is well cooked, since this will kill any of the organisms present.

The other organisms can all affect humans. Toxocara canis causes visceral larval migrans, and Giardia and Cryptosporidium can both lead to the development of diarrhoea.

13 General nursing

1. C   **The formula that should be used to determine daily basal energy requirements for animals over 5 kg is: BER (kcal) = 30 x bodyweight (in kg) + 70**

For smaller animals the formula BER (kcal) = 60 x bodyweight (in kg) should be used.

Remember that this gives *basal* energy levels. For maintenance or management of specific conditions this needs to be multiplied by a disease factor to give the animal's total energy requirement.

2. A   **The PEG tube requires the use of an endoscope for placement**

PEG actually stands for Percutaneous Endoscopically-placed Gastrostomy tube. Gastrostomy tubes can also be placed in other ways such as at surgery or using another type of introducer.

Naso-oesophageal tubes require no specific equipment for placement other than the tube itself, and enterostomy tubes require careful placement at surgery. These are not commonly used, since they tend to need elemental diets. Normal liquefied diets can be used for the other tubes.

3. C   **The only statement that is true is that water should be freely available**

In general high protein levels should be avoided, since this puts unnecessary strain on the liver and the kidneys. However, protein should still be present in the diet, and this needs to be of good quality.

Exercise is best given little and often. This gives the dog increased opportunity for urination and defaecation, and increases interest. Small walks are preferable to long ones so that the dog does not 'overdo' things, and frequent walks ensure that joints do not become too stiff through inactivity.

Often as dogs get older they become less adaptable mentally, and changes in routine can become confusing and stressful. Therefore it is always best to stick to patterns of activity that the dog expects and understands.

4. D   **The animal that is least likely to develop aspiration pneumonia is the conscious animal that is vomiting**

Conscious patients that vomit usually have full laryngeal function and this prevents the back flow of vomitus into the airways. However, in the other cases listed there is either compromise of laryngeal function, as in the anaesthetised animal, or there is a risk of there being too much food in the mouth which the animal accidentally inhales.

5. A   **It would not be appropriate to provide a paraplegic dog with a large kennel**

Paraplegic animals should be housed in a kennel that is large enough for the animal to lie out, but not so large that it could cause itself further injury by trying to drag itself about.

This is not to say that patients should not be given encouragement to walk if the veterinary surgeon is of the opinion that the animal is ready. This should be carried out under close supervision and with towels available to provide support if the animal starts to fall.

Thick padding is essential for a recumbent patient since it reduces the risk of the development of decubitus ulcers (pressure sores). Taking animals outside is also beneficial. This may help the animal urinate and defaecate naturally and improves interest. It is essential that food and water is placed within the animal's reach in the kennel. It would be immensely frustrating for an animal to be looking at its dinner, but completely unable to get to it!

6. C   **Hypostatic pneumonia can be avoided through the use of coupage 4-5 times daily**

Coupage consists of drumming on the chest with cupped hands to loosen secretions, and encourage fluid to be brought up the trachea by the ciliary carpet lining the airways. It needs to be carried out 4-5 times per day for about 5 minutes each time. Make sure that both sides of the chest are percussed.

Animals which are recumbent and are therefore at risk from hypostatic pneumonia should be turned regularly, at least every 4 hours, and where possible should be propped into sternal recumbency so that both lungs are able to function as normal.

However it is always important to check with the veterinary surgeon prior to performing any of these activities – the animal may have additional problems such as fractures that may preclude some of these techniques being used.

7. B   The catheter most suitable as an indwelling catheter in the bitch is the Foley catheter

Foley catheters can either be made of latex or silicone, and have a balloon close to their tip which is inflated by introducing a volume of water via a side port. The balloon prevents the end of the catheter slipping out of the bladder, and therefore retains it in place.

Tieman's and the metal bitch catheter can be used in the bitch, but do not stay in situ; both are for intermittent use.

Jackson's catheter is designed specifically as an indwelling catheter in the cat since the collar can be sutured in place. It is most commonly used in tom cats which are more prone to obstruction from uroliths.

8. A   Petroleum jelly should not be used as a lubricant with latex Foley catheters

The petroleum jelly can cause the latex to perish and this can cause the wall of the balloon to burst on inflation.

The other catheters are made of inert materials and there should be no problem about the type of lubricant used. However it is still more usual to use water-soluble lubricants for catheters.

9. A   Decubitus ulcers can be dressed with barrier cream

Decubitus ulcers or pressure sores are a complication of recumbency, and are difficult to manage. Prevention is therefore preferable, and regular turning of patients, the provision of thick comfortable bedding and close observation will help to reduce their incidence.

Products such as surgical spirit should not be used. In the past it was thought that these helped to harden the tissue, but they are painful and do not promote healing.

14 Medical disorders and their nursing

Infectious diseases

1. D **It is untrue that vertical transmission is transmission from a young animal to its sibling**

Vertical transmission refers to the way in which organisms are passed from parent to offspring, for example by transplacental transfer.

All the other statements are true.

There are several types of vectors – biological vectors are involved in the life cycle of the pathogen. This would therefore include intermediate hosts such as those involved in tapeworm life cycles. Mechanical vectors carry the organism unchanged. This can include the situation where the animal is able to shed the organism at any time (transport hosts), and where animals do not shed the organism, but have to be eaten for the organism to enter the final or definitive host (paratenic hosts).

Fomites are inanimate objects that act as a means of transfer of organism, and good hygiene and disinfection protocols are needed to ensure that this does not happen in the surgery.

2. C **The disease that can be described as infectious disease but not contagious is a pyometra**

In common parlance, it is very easy to be confused between infectious and contagious, but the two terms are quite different. Infection is the result of invasion by micro-organisms, and contagious refers to how the disease is spread.

Therefore sarcoptic mange is contagious but not infectious, parvovirus is both contagious and infectious, and diabetes mellitus is neither.

3. A   **An animal that has never been ill but is shedding organism is called a healthy carrier**

Convalescent carriers are those which have contracted the disease, but have now recovered, yet are still shedding organism.

Clinically affected carriers are still actually showing signs of the disease as well as actively shedding organism. These three types of carriers can also all be described as open carriers, since they are actively discharging organism.

Closed carriers have the organism within their tissues, but are not actually losing any to the environment.

4. D   **Canine distemper can lead to the development of encephalitis in older age**

In some cases where animals have apparently recovered from distemper it is possible for them to develop so-called 'old dog encephalitis' when they reach around six years of age. The disease is progressive, and the nervous signs get progressively worse until euthanasia is the only option.

5. C   **Pups from an unvaccinated mother may develop cardiac failure as a result of parvovirus infection**

Parvovirus attacks rapidly dividing cells, and in mature animals the most rapidly dividing cells are the intestinal cells. The virus damages these cells as it replicates, and this leads to the clinical signs of vomiting and diarrhoea. However, in young pups without maternal antibody protection, the virus targets the developing cells of the myocardium leading to a myocarditis. Pups present with varying degrees of heart failure – some die peracutely, whilst others show milder signs. However, the prognosis in all cases is guarded, and as the pups grow the heart muscle is less able to cope due to the permanent damage caused by the virus. Most die by the time they reach several months of age.

6. B   **The causal agent of infectious canine hepatitis is canine adenovirus 1 (CAV-1)**

Bordetella is part of the kennel cough complex and Borrelia causes Lyme disease. Leptospira icterohaemorrhagiae does affect the liver, but also affects other tissues to give a more generalised disease.

7. A   The complication that may arise after recovery from canine adenovirus 1 infection is corneal oedema

This may happen about two weeks after the initial infection. The cornea takes on a blueish colour and becomes opaque ('blue eye'). In most cases it resolves spontaneously, but in some animals there is residual scarring which shows as a white mark on the cornea.

Permanent stunting of the teeth can be the result of distemper, since the enamel organ can be damaged if the pup is infected at the time that the permanent dentition is coming through.

Malabsorption problems can be a consequence of parvovirus infection.

Liver failure is an unusual consequence after infectious disease damage. The liver has tremendous powers of recovery, and once an organism has been cleared from the animal's system it is usually able to regenerate large portions of the organ.

8. B   Leptospira canicola is potentially zoonotic

This infectious disease not only affects dogs, but also is able to affect other animals including man. Therefore everyone involved in nursing a case that is suspected of harbouring leptospira must take full care of themselves as well as minimising the risk of cross infection of other patients.

9. A   The disease caused by a bacterium is Lyme disease

Lyme disease is caused by Borrelia burgdorferi, a spirochaete. The disease is zoonotic, and is usually spread as the result of the deer tick carrying the infection from deer to other species including dogs and humans.

All the other diseases listed are viral in origin.

10. C Distemper may lead to the development of respiratory signs in affected animals

Distemper is a complex disease which may present with a number of different signs including respiratory signs, vomiting and diarrhoea, nervous signs, damage to the teeth, hyperkeratosis of the pads and nasal skin, and skin rashes. This makes it quite difficult to diagnose, since for each presentation there are other organisms that produce a similar clinical picture.

11. D Chlamydia psittaci usually leads to conjunctivitis and chemosis, and occasionally causes abortion in the pregnant queen

This is the same organism that causes psittacosis in birds, but is a different strain, and is considered not to be zoonotic (unlike the bird form).

12. C At present there is no vaccine against feline infectious peritonitis in the UK

On the continent vaccines are being used, but the protection rate is not yet good enough to be acceptable in this country. Therefore there is no good way of specifically protecting against this disease.

All the other diseases listed have effective vaccines, though the chlamydia vaccine is probably the least long lasting.

13. A The most common FeLV associated disease is lymphosarcoma

About 15% of persistently viraemic animals present with one of the forms of lymphosarcoma.

The other diseases listed are all possible developments in an animal infected with FeLV, but each represents only a small percentage of the total number of cases.

14. A The cats most likely to become persistently infected with FeLV are kittens infected in utero

All kittens infected at this stage in their development will remain viraemic, and will die.

Kittens infected whilst their immune system is developing (under 8 weeks) are also highly likely to remain infected, and will therefore develop clinical signs at some stage. Animals infected after the immune system has matured are far more likely to fight off the infection (only about 10% remain viraemic), but it is important to note that these animals may still harbour a latent infection, and could therefore still be a threat to other cats.

15. B   Antibody-antigen complexes form in feline infectious peritonitis and lead to a vasculitis

The clinical signs seen in FIP infections depend where these complexes are deposited and what effect this has on the tissues. If they cause a vasculitis in the thorax or abdomen, then free fluid accumulates within the body cavities, giving rise to the 'wet form' of FIP. However if they are deposited in other areas where there is no space for an effusion, for example in the cerebral vascular system, they cause signs associated with damage to that organ. This is usually referred to as the 'dry form' of FIP.

16. C   The best advice to give an owner of a well FIV-infected cat, would be to keep the cat indoors away from other cats until it falls ill

Once the animal develops clinical signs and its quality of life deteriorates it should be euthanased.

Occasionally this is not possible – the temperament of the cat could make this too stressful for the animal and owner, or the client has other cats that are FIV negative, and this would therefore pose too great a risk. In these cases euthanasia may need to be considered.

Animals infected with FIV do not get better and throw off the virus, and although the organism does not last long outside of the host it is sensible to ensure that contact between cats is not possible if one has the virus.

17. D   Feline calici virus does not show latency

Organisms that become latent are able to 'hide' within the animal's body, and can remain there without causing clinical signs. However, stress may cause the virus to be reactivated, for active shedding to recur, and the redevelopment of clinical signs.

Animals that have been infected with calici virus may remain carriers, but they shed continuously throughout the time that the organism is present.

18. A **Canine parvovirus is closely related to feline panleucopaenia**

Feline panleucopaenia (also called feline infectious enteritis) is caused by a parvovirus, and in 1978 this is thought to have mutated to the canine form and canine parvovirus infections were seen for the first time.

Non-infectious diseases

19. C **The administration of oxygen via a tent made from a buster collar and cling film may lead to hyperthermia if an animal is panting excessively**

Oxygen cages may also lead to the same problem.

Masks are quick and easy to use, but are often poorly tolerated by the patients.

Flow by techniques can be quite easy to use, but generally give a lower level of oxygenation than other methods.

Nasal tubes, although more difficult to place, can be very effective for longterm oxygen therapy.

20. D **All the signs described may be seen in an animal with laryngeal paralysis**

21. B **Endocardiosis is a cardiac disease that is not congenital**

Endocardiosis occurs in older animals, and is the result of the formation of nodules on the cusps of valves. This leads to valvular incompetence – particularly of the atrio-ventricular valves which will in time lead to heart failure. There is no corrective treatment, so drugs are used simply to manage the disease.

The other problems are congenital. Patent ductus arteriosus is a condition that arises in young animals when the duct does not close as it should after birth. A shunt remains between the aorta and pulmonary artery, and left-sided heart failure may develop.

A ventricular septal defect is literally a 'hole in the heart' – a gap in the wall between the two ventricles. Surgery is possible, but not always carried out, depending on the degree of the problem.

Tetralogy of Fallot is a rare congenital defect. It is made up of 3 congenital defects – pulmonic stenosis, ventricular septal defect and an over-riding aorta. These result in heart failure, despite the heart trying to cope by hypertrophy of the right ventricle (often described as the fourth defect).

22. D Nitroglycerine ointment is used in the treatment of acute heart failure as it is a venodilator and reduces the heart's workload by lowering blood pressure

Nitroglycerine is generally used as an ointment spread on the inside of the pinna. Gloves should always be worn when handling this medication.

Diuretics are used to reduce circulating blood volume, again to make it easier for the heart to cope.

Other drugs may be used at the discretion of the clinician, but this will vary depending on the reason for the heart failure.

23. B Polycythaemia does not lead to anaemia

Remember, anaemia is a clinical sign, not an actual condition. Anaemia is strictly defined as a lack of haemoglobin, – often this also means a lack of red blood cells (but not always).

Polycythaemia is a rare condition in which excessive numbers of red blood cells are produced, and the blood becomes more viscous than normal. This makes it harder for the heart to pump, and consequently can lead to signs of heart failure.

Iron deficiency means that normal amounts of haemoglobin cannot be produced, since iron is essential for the haem part of the molecule.

Chronic renal failure can also lead to anaemia since erythropoietin, produced by the kidney, is needed for red cell production and maturation.

Von Willebrand's disease is a clotting disorder, and animals with this condition are often slightly anaemic since small bleeds which occur every day through knocks and bumps are obviously more serious in these patients.

24. B The description that could be applied to true vomiting is that the animal usually starts to salivate, and then abdominal contractions start before the animal brings up partially digested food

The description given in A refers to pharyngeal retching.

That given in C describes regurgitation. This is a passive process, and the animal makes no effort to bring up the food, it simply falls out!

25. D **Key-Gaskell syndrome (feline dysautonomia) would not lead to an animal developing diarrhoea**

This condition results when the parasympathetic nervous supply to the gastrointestinal tract fails to function properly, and normal gut tone is lost. The colon often becomes enlarged and flaccid; faeces accumulate within it, and are not passed normally.

Diarrhoea is a common sign seen in the other conditions listed, either due to maldigestion or malabsorption of the nutrients.

26. A **The least appropriate advice is to do nothing**

For many fit animals this might be fine, but it is not good professional advice. It is best to see if the problem will sort itself out by resting the stomach, just giving small amounts of water little and often rather than continuing to challenge the animal with food.

If after 24 hours there has been no vomiting, then the next step is to continue on a bland, easily digestible diet. However, if there is no improvement then the dog should be seen.

27. B **The signs of an animal passing faeces frequently, often with blood and mucus, is suggestive of a large intestinal problem rather than a small intestinal problem**

The other signs are usually linked to small intestinal causes of diarrhoea.

An animal that is eating well, but shows weight loss and diarrhoea should be checked for malabsorption or maldigestion problems.

Broborygmi means intestinal gurgles and rumbles, and this is more usually seen with small intestine diseases.

Tenesmus means straining, and it is more common to see straining with large intestinal problems such as colitis where the animal feels increased urgency to defaecate although the actual volumes passed are not necessarily very large.

28. C   **The post-renal cause of acute renal failure is bladder rupture**

In renal failure, the body is unable to clear nitrogenous waste from the bloodstream. In pre-renal cases this is due to insufficient blood flow to and through the renal tissues, so the blood is not filtered properly.

Renal causes such as ethylene glycol toxicity or leptospirosis actually damage the renal tubules so that they are unable to function normally. Post-renal problems prevent the urine from leaving the body, so urinary obstructions or ruptures would come into this category.

29. A   **Hyperadrenocorticism can be tested for using a low dose dexamethasone screening test**

Hyperadrenocorticism (Cushing's disease) results in abnormally high levels of plasma cortisol. Normally if animals are given intravenous dexamethasone then their natural levels of cortisol should drop as the adrenal gland is suppressed. However, in cases of Cushing's disease this does not occur.

30. D   **Hyperparathyroidism can lead to reduced bone density and the development of spontaneous fractures**

Primary hyperparathyroidism is quite rare, but when it does occur, there is increased bone resorption, and the bones become very fragile. Blood calcium levels rise and this can cause problems with nerve and muscle function.

Increased appetite and weight loss are associated with hyperthyroidism.

Hypocalcaemia, muscle spasm and rigidity could be due to hypoparathyroidism – usually the result of accidental removal or bruising after thyroidectomies in cats. Alternatively, hypocalcaemia can be due to eclampsia in bitches.

Bilateral symmetrical alopecia occurs in a number of hormonal conditions such as hypothyroidism, Cushing's disease, lack of growth hormone, and abnormalities in the levels of the sex hormones oestrogen and testosterone.

31. B   The term that relates to unilateral paralysis is hemiplegia

Quadriplegia and tetraplagia both refer to cases in which all four limbs are paralysed, and paraplegia refers to an animal paralysed in the hind limbs only.

32. D   Hypertrophic osteodystrophy develops as a result of the presence of intra-thoracic or intra-abdominal masses

This is an odd condition, most commonly seen due to space-occupying lesions in the thoracic cavity. The long bones of the limbs become inflamed and painful, so the animal shows shifting lameness. Unless the mass can be removed there is no cure, just pain management. If the mass is excised then the skeletal signs resolve spontaneously.

Rickets is rare, but can occur due to lack of calcium or vitamin D in the diet. It can also be the result of lack of sunlight, since ingested vitamin D requires activation in the skin through interaction with UV light.

Metaphyseal osteopathy is a disease of young dogs, and affects the regions close to the growth plates – the metaphyses. These become swollen and inflamed, and the animal shows lameness. The animals usually grow out of the condition as they get older, but the cause is not fully understood.

Osteochondrosis is a very complex disease of the joints in which the articular cartilage fails to develop normally. There are three forms – osteochondrosis is the mildest, osteochondritis is worse, and the most severe is osteochondritis dissecans (OCD). There is a genetic component to its cause, which is why there is now an Elbow Scheme, in which screening radiographs are used to identify animals with the problem before they are bred from. However, nutrition is also thought to play a role, and pups from susceptible breeds should not be pushed to grow too fast.

33. C   Oestrogen, if present in large amounts, can lead to bone marrow suppression

This can be a problem in dogs with Sertoli cell tumours, and is the reason that female cats cannot be given oestrodiol benzoate in cases of mismating. Cats have a far greater oestrogen sensitivity than dogs.

34. D **Urticaria is the term used to describe an acute allergic reaction in which the animal develops multiple small pruritic swellings in the skin**

Urticaria can develop as the result of insect bites or plant stings, for example nettles.

Atopic dermatitis is also an allergic condition, but this usually leads to intense irritation without the development of swellings. It is usually associated with the face, feet, axilla and ventral abdomen.

Impetigo is a form of pyoderma usually seen in puppies where small pustules develop on the ventral abdomen or under the chin. Usually the pups grow out of this as they get older, but it can be managed by the use of antiseptics and antibacterial shampoos.

Furunculosis is also a pyoderma, but is far more serious. This is an invasive pyoderma and deep fistulae develop. It can be very debilitating, and surgery, cryotherapy and longterm antibiotics can be used. Prognosis should always be guarded as there may be other underlying disease.

35. C **Intradermal skin testing can be used to test for atopic dermatitis**

In this form of testing, animals are challenged with suspect allergens by injecting tiny quantities of each into the skin, and observing the sites for reaction. These are compared with reaction from histamine and sterile saline (the positive and negative controls). Often animals are allergic to a number of allergens, and management regimes should then be introduced to minimise exposure to these.

Dietary hypersensitivity is tested for by the use of exclusion diets which contain novel protein and carbohydrate sources.

Contact dermatitis can be tested for through the use of patch tests – very similar to those used for human allergy sufferers. Alternatively contact elimination can be used, but this involves taking the animal out of its normal environment and keeping it hospitalised until signs resolve, so that challenge can then be made with specific items.

Urticaria is not usually tested for, since this leads to sporadic one-off problems, and usually resolves without longterm problems.

15 Obstetric and paediatric nursing of the dog and cat

1. C **Under the Sale of Goods Act, owners of breeding animals have to ensure that pups or kittens sold are clinically healthy and have a sound temperament**

The Breeding and Sale of Dogs Act is designed to ensure the welfare of the bitch and pups during the time they are with the breeder.

Protection of Animals Acts also relate primarily to welfare issues, and list what constitutes a cruelty offence.

The Trade Description Act does not relate to the sale of animals.

2. C **Testes should have descended in the male dog by 10 days after birth**

In tom cats, the testes descend earlier, and are usually in the scrotum at birth.

3. B **Cryptorchidism is the term used to describe the condition in which one or both testes are retained within the abdomen**

Anorchia is very rare – this is the absence of both testes.

Monorchidism is also rare – this occurs when an animal only develops one testis. (Occasionally this term is used incorrectly to describe a cryptorchid animal, in which there is one retained testis.)

Orchitis is inflammation of the testes.

4. B **The fraction of the canine ejaculate that contains the sperm is the second fraction**

The first fraction mainly consists of a clear fluid from the prostate. The third fraction is also prostatic in origin, and it is thought that its function is to flush the sperm through the cervix and on into the uterus.

5. D **Metoestrus in the bitch usually lasts about 55 days**

This is the stage of progesterone dominance and is the time during which the corpora lutea are active.

Pro-oestrus and oestrus last for about 7 days each (though this can be quite variable), and anoestrus lasts 4 months on average. The total oestrous cycle is therefore approximately 7 months. However, not all bitches follow these timings precisely.

6. D **The queen is an induced ovulator and a seasonal breeder**

The bitch, on the other hand, is the opposite – she is a spontaneous ovulator and a non-seasonal breeder.

7. A **Blood tests used to detect oestrus in the bitch test for the presence of progesterone**

Prior to ovulation there is very little progesterone in the bloodstream, but once ovulation has occurred and the corpus luteum is formed then progesterone is released.

Therefore blood samples should be tested from several days before ovulation is anticipated, and as soon as progesterone is detected the animal should be mated.

8. B **Animals which have both male and female genital tissue are described as intersexes**

These animals have features of both sexes, but are not true hermaphrodites and certainly cannot self fertilise. In fact they are usually sterile with neither type of genital tissue functioning.

9. D   **Of the methods of pregnancy diagnosis listed, ultrasound can be used earliest in the bitch**

Ultrasound can be carried out as early as 16 days after ovulation, but usually tests are carried out around 28 days for maximum accuracy.

Abdominal palpation can be carried out after a month, but not all animals will allow the veterinary surgeon to feel, as they may tense the abdominal wall muscles.

Identification of foetal heart beats is only possible in late pregnancy, as is radiography. Radiographic techniques may show a swollen, enlarged uterus earlier in pregnancy, but it is not until the foetal skeletons start to ossify that it is possible to distinguish pregnancy from a pyometra.

In addition to the tests suggested, hormone assay testing for the hormone relaxin can now be used in both species.

10. A   **The statement that the term foetus describes the developing young from day 10 after ovulation is incorrect**

The term embryo should be used for the young animal until discernable features are present (about day 35) and then the word foetus can be used.

The definitions for resorption, abortion and stillbirth are correct.

11. C   **The temperature of the area in which the bitch is due to whelp should be maintained at 25-30°C**

This can be reduced several days after the pups have been born since the bitch will find this very warm, and the pups will start to be able to thermoregulate.

12. A   **A rise in body temperature of about 2°C is not a sign of imminent parturition**

There is usually a *drop* in temperature of about 2°C about 24-36 hours before parturition. The other signs described are also likely to occur in the time preceding the first delivery.

13. D   Breech birth is a cause of foetal dystocia

Dystocia means difficulty giving birth, and the terms foetal and maternal are used to indicate with which individual the problem lies.

A breech birth occurs when a pup or kitten is presented rump first. Posterior presentations, when the hindlegs come through the pelvic canal first, are not breech, and these are normally delivered without problem.

Uterine inertia simply means that the uterus fails to contract. This can be a primary problem, or may be secondary to other problems such as hypocalcaemia or exhaustion.

Obstructive dystocias develop when there is a physical obstruction to the birth canal caused by either bony deformities (e.g. an old fracture to the pelvis) or soft tissue problems (e.g. vaginal polyps).

Thus uterine inertia, obstructive dystocia and exhaustion are all maternal dystocias, since in each case the problem is due to the mother.

14. C   Pups are normally able to stand from about 10 days of age

However, they are not fully able to walk until they are 3 weeks old. Other developmental changes that take a while to happen include the opening of ears and eyes which occurs at about 10-14 days of age. Kittens are often born with a squint, or strabismus, which usually self corrects by the time the kittens are about 8 weeks old. However, Siamese cats may retain this characteristic into adulthood.

15. D   The puerperium usually lasts about 6 weeks

The puerperium is the period of time after the end of parturition during which the uterus involutes and returns to an inactive state.

16. B   Placental retention might be identifiable clinically by the presence of a persistent green vulval discharge

Normally after parturition there is a bloody discharge for

about a week, and this then becomes clear whilst the uterus involutes.

However, with a retained placenta the green-coloured discharge seen prior to birth continues, and if left untreated, the bitch or queen may go on to develop a metritis.

Diagnosis is confirmed by ultrasound or palpation, and if detected can be treated with oxytocin. This encourages the expulsion of the remaining placenta.

17. D   The dam normally needs to stimulate urination and defaecation in neonatal pups or kittens for 2-3 weeks after birth

This is an important consideration when dealing with orphan pups or kittens, since they too will require this attention. Therefore gentle wiping of the anogenital area with warm moistened cotton wool is required after each feeding.

18. B   Polydactyly poses no threat to the animal's health

Polydactyly is simply the presence of extra digits, and is not uncommon in cats.

Atresia ani occurs when the anal opening does not form, so faeces cannot be passed.

Cleft palate is a failure of the fusion of the two halves of the hard palate, so that a pup or kitten is unable to suck normally, and if it does manage to get some milk, this often comes back down the nostrils.

An open fontanelle occurs when the bones of the skull do not fuse properly, leaving a hole in the cranium. If this does not close, it leaves the young animal prone to brain damage.

16 Surgical and high-dependence nursing

1. D   **Pus is not a cardinal sign of inflammation**

There are five signs described as 'cardinal' signs: heat, redness, swelling, pain and loss of normal function. These are present in all cases of inflammation regardless of cause.

Pus may be present in some inflammatory conditions, but is certainly not present in all.

2. C   **The fluid formed as a result of inflammation that contains white cells and proteinaceous debris is exudate**

Transudate is fluid that has passed across a semipermeable membrane, and is therefore acellular, for example the ascitic fluid formed in the abdomen in hypoproteinaemia.

Modified transudate describes a transudate that also contains some inflammatory cells since it has started to cause an inflammatory reaction in its own right.

Chyle is simply the fluid that should be within the lymphatic system.

3. B   **Surgical removal of the gall bladder is termed a cholecystectomy**

Celiotomy is another term used to describe a laparotomy or temporary opening into the abdomen.

Orchidectomy means surgical removal of the testes (castration), and tenotomy refers to the surgical procedure of splitting a tendon.

4. A   **A fresh open wound should be considered to be contaminated but not infected for a maximum of 6 hours**

After this time bacterial multiplication starts to become more significant, and by the time the wound is over 12 hours old, bacterial invasion of the tissues is taking place, and the wound is therefore 'dirty'.

5. D   **The clipper blade that should be used for the final clip prior to surgery is a No. 40 blade**

If the coat is very coarse it may be appropriate to use a No. 10 blade initially, but for a sufficiently fine final cut the No. 40 should still be used.

If the practice sees a number of exotic species it may be worth investing in smaller high-speed clippers since the coat is finer and the skin thinner in these animals.

Care should always be taken not to damage the skin, and not to allow the clippers to become too hot.

6. C   **The minimum margin suggested for clipping and prepping is 15 cm from the incision site**

This is to ensure that there is no contamination of the incision site by hair during the operation. However, there will obviously be variation depending on the type and location of the procedure.

7. B   **Post-operative bandages should be changed 24 hours after application**

This is to allow examination of the affected area, and to prevent pressure problems if the tissues swell after the operation.

8. A   **0.5% chlorhexidine solution is suitable for lavage of a contaminated wound**

Note that even this solution is toxic to fibroblasts. The only completely safe solutions are isotonic solutions such as sterile 0.9% saline or Hartmann's solution, but these have no antibacterial activity.

Hydrogen peroxide has been used in the past for flushing abscesses, but this damages healthy cells, and remains an irritant for 4-5 days after use.

Savlon, commonly used in the home, is also not to be recommended since this combination (cetrimide + cetavlon) is very toxic to cells as well as being an irritant.

Hypochlorite solutions are bleach solutions, which are toxic and irritant to cells and should therefore be avoided.

9. C   Alginate dressings stimulate the production of granulation tissue, and can be used to control low level haemorrhage

These are seaweed-based products that interact with the wound surface and release either sodium or calcium to stimulate inflammation and promote wound healing.

Saline-soaked swabs are wet when placed, but gradually dry out so that when they are removed the top layers of cells are removed from the wound. This can be a useful technique to debride certain wounds in the early stage of their management. They are sometimes referred to as wet-to-dry dressings.

Paraffin gauze dressings are non-adherent, and are used if a water impermeable layer is required immediately over the wound. This can be useful for burn management.

Hydrogel dressings are useful when there is some healthy granulation tissue, but there are still areas that require debridement, since the dressing will not harm the healthy new tissue.

10. C   For free skin grafts the bandage *should* be left on for 5-7 days

This is to avoid interference with the wound and to prevent damage to the fragile vascular supply that is (hopefully) starting to form.

It is true that if the graft bed was inadequately prepared, the graft was able to move slightly, or serum or haemorrhage accumulated under the graft, there is likely to be graft failure.

11. A   **Aloe vera ointment actively stimulates the development of granulation tissue**

This is only true if the product chosen contains a very pure extract.

Malic, benzoic and salicylic acid solution (Dermisol) is very acidic and is used as a debriding agent. Therefore this would damage developing granulation tissue.

Zinc bacitracin ointment enhances epithelialisation, and silver sulphadiazine ointment (Flamazine) is good for preventing infection and sepsis relating to burns.

12. D   **The fracture that could be treated using an external coaption technique is the spiral fracture of the tibia**

Fractures can only be managed by external fixation methods if two criteria are fulfilled – the fracture must be distal to the elbow or stifle, since the support must fix the joint both above and below the fracture, and the fracture must be stable.

The first point rules out the management of femoral or scapular fractures by this method. Transverse fractures are not stable since the fragments are able to rotate, even within a cast or heavy bandage. Therefore these too require a different type of management.

13. B   **It is untrue that only some types of fractures can be managed by internal fixation**

With appropriate equipment, any type of fracture can be repaired using internal fixation techniques

The other statements are true.

14. C   **The parallel sided plate with 4 to 8 round screw holes is the Venables plate**

Both Sherman and Lane plates also have round holes, but these are not parallel sided. The metal narrows between each screw hole to reduce the weight of the plate. Lane plates are small and relatively weak. Sherman plates are stronger, but are still less so than the Venables plate.

The dynamic compression plate or DCP is a more highly

engineered plate which has shaped screw holes that appear oval when looking down onto the plate. Depending on the placement of the screws, these can be used to compress the fracture site and reduce any gap that might exist between the fracture fragments. This tends to give better and faster fracture healing.

15. B   It is true that fracture disease may develop if external coaption methods have been used to stabilise a fracture

External coaption methods include casts, splints and support bandages, and there are several potential problems with their use.

Pressure sores and cast loosening are quite common, as is fracture disease, where the restriction in the use of the limb causes the joints to stiffen and muscles to atrophy. In severe cases the joint can become fibrosed, and the range of movement is permanently restricted.

No implant is used, therefore osteomyelitis and reactions to implants are not a consequence of external coaption techniques.

16. D   An allograft is a bone graft taken from a different animal of the same species

Bone grafts may be needed to pack around fracture sites where there is substantial bone tissue loss. The graft acts as a scaffold on which new bone may form. Once the animal produces its own bone in the location, osteoclasts gradually break down the 'foreign' bone since its job is now done.

17. B   Luxation of the patella is commonly the result of congenital problems

In congenital patella luxations the trochlear groove is quite shallow, and the patella is able to slip off medially. The joint capsule becomes stretched and loose, and recurrence becomes more frequent.

Hip, elbow and carpal luxations are usually traumatic in origin, and there may be tremendous soft tissue disruption with these.

18. D   Melanomas are very often malignant tumours

This is particularly true if they form within the oral cavity. The other tumours listed are all benign tumours.

19. A   It is true that sarcomas are malignant tumours of connective tissue

There are two main types of malignant tumours – sarcomas and carcinomas. Carcinomas form from epithelial tissue.

The prefix adeno- always relates to glandular tissue, so adenomas are benign tumours of a gland.

Fibrosarcomas are malignant tumours of fibroblasts and can be found in any connective tissue.

20. C   A gastrotomy would be classed as a clean-contaminated procedure

Procedures can be divided into four categories:

i.   clean procedures in which there is no break in aseptic conditions, such as repair of an umbilical hernia

ii. clean-contaminated procedures where a body cavity is entered but there is no spillage, for example a gastrotomy

iii. contaminated procedures where there is a spill from a viscus, or break in sterile technique such as repair of wounds less than 4 hours old, or lower bowel surgery

iv. dirty procedures where there is known to be infection, for example oral surgery or abscess treatment.

21. C   Keratitis is inflammation of the cornea

Corneal inflammation causes the cornea to become opaque, often taking on a bluish colouration.

Inflammation of the skin is dermatitis.

Overflow of tears is described as epiphora and inflammation of the eyelids is bleparitis.

22. A   Left untreated, glaucoma can lead to permanent damage to the retina and blindness

Glaucoma describes a condition in which the intraocular pressure is raised due to lack of drainage of the aqueous humour. This may be the result of either an inherited problem, or trauma.

Distichiasis is an extra row of eyelashes which irritate the surface of the cornea causing a keratitis and epiphora. It has no effect on the retina.

Cataracts are opacities which develop within or on the lens. Superficial or capsular cataracts can be removed to leave a functional lens, but nuclear cataracts in the centre of the lens cannot. In all cases sight becomes progressively blurred until no light gets through. The retina is not actually damaged.

Corneal foreign bodies will cause similar but more localised signs to those seen in distichiasis. It is important that the foreign body is removed as quickly as possible to prevent the development of further ulceration.

23. D   It is not true that mammary tumours in the cat are usually benign

Over 80% of mammary tumours in the cat are malignant, so any masses detected should be excised with a good margin as soon as they are detected. In the bitch about 50% of the growths are malignant.

The use of drains post-operatively is to be advised since this reduces the risk of tension on the sutures and wound breakdown.

Mastectomies involve the removal of at least two glands with radical mastectomies being full 'mammary strips'; all of the glands on one side are removed, whereas in a mammectomy just one gland is excised.

24. B   The extraction of canine teeth can result in the development of an oronasal fistula

In small animals the canine teeth have relatively long roots compared with the depth of bone, and it is not difficult to get the formation of an oronasal fistula between oral and nasal cavities when the tooth is removed. This should be repaired surgically to ensure that food is not pushed into the nasal cavity where it would cause a rhinitis.

25. B   The most appropriate solution to use as a mouthwash for animals is 0.2% chlorhexidine solution

Hydrogen peroxide and hypochlorite (bleach) solutions would be dangerous to use. Povidone-iodine could be used, but the concentration would need to be far lower – 0.1% would be appropriate.

26. C   A gastrostomy tube should be left in place for 5 days before removal

This is to ensure that a seal has formed around the ostomy site, and no leakage of stomach contents into the abdominal cavity can occur.

After removal there may be leakage from the fistula to the outside for a few days, but this will then seal over quite quickly.

27. D   Bronchial inflammation does not contribute to the brachycephalic airway obstruction syndrome

BAOS mainly relates to upper airway problems, and includes stenotic nares, foreshortened nasal chambers, overlong soft palate and hypoplastic trachea. Tonsillar hypertrophy and laryngeal collapse are often seen as secondary changes.

28. A   Gynaecomastia is the sign in a male dog that is suggestive of a Sertoli cell tumour

Sertoli cells in the testes normally secrete nutrients for the developing sperm, and small amounts of oestrogen. If a tumour develops within this cell type, oestrogen is released in larger quantities and some degree of feminisation may take place, including the development of the mammary glands – gynaecomastia.

There may also be hair loss, atrophy of the other testis, and if oestrogen levels become very high, bone marrow suppression and anaemia.

Anal adenomas and male libido are both testosterone dependent, and therefore would not increase in this condition.

29. B   A rupture in which the contents become devitalised due to compression of the blood vessels supplying them is described as strangulated

Incarcerated or irreducible ruptures are those which have contents that cannot be replaced by manipulation alone, usually due to the formation of adhesions.

The contents of a reducible rupture can be gently massaged back into the correct part of the body (usually the abdomen).

30. A   An arthrodesis would be carried out in order to surgically fuse a joint and prevent its movement

Arthroscopy involves the use of an arthroscope to visualise the internal structures of a joint.

Arthrotomy simply describes an operation in which there is an incision made into a joint cavity. It does not describe the procedure in any more depth.

Arthropexy is not a term used in orthopaedic surgery.

31. C   Treatments such as intravenous and urinary catheters can contribute to the development of nosocomial infection

Nosocomial infection is infection resulting from an animal's stay in the hospital kennel, and is usually associated with poor hygiene techniques or other disease processes lowering the animal's resistance to infection.

However it can also be linked to treatments which are apparently doing the animal good, such as the use of intravenous fluid therapy or an indwelling urinary catheter. It can even be associated with antibiotic use if that treatment is over-zealous and not specific.

32. A   The least reactive material to be made into urinary catheters is silicone

Silicone is being used for catheters more widely now, since it is very inert, and causes minimal irritation to the mucosa of the urethra.

All the other materials can cause some tissue reaction which will increase the risk of infection.

33. B   If a pulse oximeter is to be used during patient monitoring, oxygen saturation levels should remain above 93%

If the level falls below this, then additional oxygen therapy should be started.

34. C   It is possible to measure blood pressure through the use of an arterial catheter connected to a manometer

However this technique is quite invasive and therefore rarely carried out.

Peripheral pulses provide very useful information about the circulation and how well the blood is reaching the periphery. However, blood pressure is not actually assessed using this technique – the pulse is merely the difference between systolic and diastolic pressures.

The most accurate way of measuring blood pressure using non-invasive techniques is via the use of Doppler systems; oscillometric systems are easy to use, but not as reliable in small patients.

Central venous pressure can only be measured if a vein such as the jugular is used, since the catheter needs to be long and placed such that its tip lies in or very close to the vena cava. This is not possible with peripheral veins such as the cephalic or saphenous veins.

35. D   Transcutaneous electrical nerve stimulation (TENS) can be used to provide some pain relief

The other physiotherapy techniques listed can all provide benefit to patients after injury or surgery, but need to be used carefully under veterinary direction. There are specific indications and contraindications for each.

36. C **Total parenteral nutrition is supplied by feeding via an intravenous line**

The term parenteral refers to the giving of a drug or food via a route that does not involve the gastrointestinal tract. Naso-gastric and oesophagostomy tubes obviously enter the stomach and oesophagus respectively, and PEG tubes are a form of gastrostomy tube (Percutaneous Endoscopically-placed Gastrostomy tubes), and are therefore placed into the stomach.

17 Theatre practice

1. A   Asepsis is the absence of micro-organisms and spores

Disinfection also refers to the destruction of micro-organisms, but the difference between this and sterilisation is that the latter also removes or destroys bacterial spores. This is not guaranteed with disinfection. The term antisepsis is used when a disinfectant is used on skin or living tissue, not the environment.

Sterilisation can be achieved using heat methods as described, but also through the use of chemicals such as ethylene oxide, or by radiation.

2. D   Repair of a fresh wound to the thigh region would be classed as a contaminated procedure

As described in the surgical nursing section, surgical procedures can be classed into 4 categories:

Clean procedures – where no contaminated body systems are entered, such as the closed fracture.

Clean-contaminated – where a contaminated system is entered, but there is no spillage, such as the gastrotomy.

Contaminated – where there is spillage from a contaminated system, or there is severe inflammation, such as a fresh clean traumatic wound.

Dirty – where there is infection or devitalised tissue, or a traumatic wound contains foreign bodies, such as the infected bite wound.

3. C   The colour of the fluid in Browne's tube changes from red to green during the sterilising process

Different Browne's tubes are available for different temperature and time combinations. They can therefore be used in both autoclaves and hot air ovens. Note that they do not detect steam, and therefore are probably not the best indicator to use in an autoclave.

4. D   Sterilisation of instruments in a hot air oven operating at 150°C takes 180 minutes

The cutting edges of sharp instruments are dulled by very high heat levels, so it is usual for a temperature at the lower end of the hot air oven's range to be used in order to prolong instrument life. This does mean a longer sterilising time compared with materials such as glass which can be sterilised at 180°C for 60 minutes. However, hot air ovens are considered to be better than autoclaves for very fine ophthalmic instruments and glassware, and for materials such as powders and oils which cannot be steam sterilised.

5. B   It is untrue that open shelves are the best means for storing equipment in theatre

There are two problems with this statement – open shelves are actually a poor way of storing equipment since they easily harbour dust. Closed cabinets are therefore preferable. However, it is better still to have no equipment actually stored in theatre. Surgical packs and other theatre equipment should be stored adjacent to theatre in a dedicated storage cupboard.

6. C   Surgical masks should be changed between every procedure

Surgical masks prevent micro-organisms from the wearer's mouth and nose entering the environment, but are only effective for quite short periods of time. Therefore they should be changed regularly. It would be inappropriate to change them during a procedure; best practise is that they should be changed between each operation.

7. B   It is untrue that clipping over 12 hours before surgery reduces the number of skin bacteria

Studies have found that clipping this far in advance of surgery may actually increase the number of skin bacteria, thereby making it harder to achieve asepsis.

Also, be aware that clipping just before surgery increases the risk of infection, since it is very difficult, even with hand-held vacuum cleaners, to remove all the loose hairs before surgery commences.

8. D   Esmarch's bandage is used in conjunction with a tourniquet to create a bloodless surgical field

It is a rubber bandage which is applied tightly to a distal limb, in order to push blood back into more central vessels. A tourniquet is then applied, and Esmarch's bandage then removed. The operation may then take place with minimal haemorrhage. However, tourniquets should not be left in place for longer than 15-20 minutes. The procedures for which this may be useful include digit amputation or investigation of foreign body sinuses.

9. C   Instrument cleaning solutions containing enzymes may be used

All the other statements are untrue.

Instruments should be cleaned under cool or luke-warm water. Hot water coagulates proteins and makes them harder to remove.

Ratchets and box joints of instruments placed in an ultrasonic bath should be left open.

Abrasive powders should not be used since these will damage the instruments.

10. B   The scalpel blade with a fine straight cutting edge, sometimes referred to as a tenotomy blade, is size 11

Scalpel blade sizes 10 and 15 are most commonly used in small animal practice for general surgery. Size 15 is the smaller of the two, and may be preferred for surgery of smaller species. A size 12 blade has a small, scythe-like cutting edge, and can be used for suture removal.

11. A   Sutures can be removed post-operatively using Pains scissors

The other three types of scissors are all used intra-operatively. Metzenbaum and Mayo scissors are both surgical scissors used for the dissection of tissues. Carless scissors are specifically for cutting sutures during operations, and are used in order to conserve the blades of the dissecting scissors.

12. B   The Balfour retractor would be suitable to retract the abdominal wall

Gelpi, Travers and West's retractors are all relatively small, and usually used to retract muscle or joint tissue. The key difference between them is the tips of the retractors since each has a different number of prongs. The Balfour retractor is far larger and provides means not only for lateral retraction, but also for retraction in a cranial or caudal direction.

13. A   It is true that ASIF equipment is more highly engineered and allows fractures to be repaired more precisely

It is expensive equipment, and there are plates and screws designed for many different types of orthopaedic procedure. The most common plate used is the Dynamic Compression Plate. This has holes that have been designed to allow the placement of screws so that the two fracture fragments are brought closer together as the screws are tightened.

All ASIF equipment is measured in millimetres.

14. D   The most suitable means of sterilising a fibre-optic flexible endoscope would be ethylene oxide

In day-to-day use, endoscopes are usually cleaned thoroughly and disinfected rather than actually sterilised. However if there is risk of infection, then sterilisation should be considered. Glutaraldehyde solutions have been used in the past, but this takes a long time (soaking for 24 hours) and the instrument should be rinsed thoroughly with sterile water or saline before use.

Ethylene oxide is also a slow technique, but after sterilisation and airing, the endoscope is guaranteed to be sterile and ready for use. Practices using ethylene oxide, however, must adhere to the safety procedures, since it is a very toxic product.

15. D   The tendency of a suture material to coil back into its original packaged shape is described as memory

There are many words used to describe suture materials.

Drag describes the frictional force generated as a suture is pulled through a tissue. Capillarity describes how easily fluid is drawn along the length of the material. Chatter refers to the lack of smoothness as a knot is tightened and the two strands of the knot slide over each other. Braided sutures show all these features, whereas monofilament materials are more likely to show memory.

16. B Polyamide is a non-absorbable suture material

The other products listed are all absorbable. All of the products are synthetic polymers, as their names suggest.

17. A The suture material removed from the operation site by phagocytosis is catgut

All natural absorbable products will be removed from the body by this method. It does, however, result in some tissue reaction and this may lead to wound breakdown in some instances.

Synthetic absorbable products such as polyglactin 910 are removed by hydrolysis (enzymatic breakdown in the presence of water) which causes less reaction.

Both the polyesters and linen are non-absorbable.

Note that catgut may no longer be in use due to EC regulations.

18. A The continuous suture pattern suitable for skin closure is the Ford interlocking suture pattern

Whilst suitable for skin closure, the other patterns listed are all interrupted patterns. Which pattern is chosen depends on the surgeon's preference, and the degree of tension on the sutures.

19. C The smallest suture material listed is 6/0

Metric sizes are quite straightforward to use: to get the actual diameter of the thread, simply divide the number by 10. Thus a 3 metric suture has a diameter of 0.3 mm.

The USP system is more complicated – smaller sutures are described as x/0, where the number x gets larger as the suture gets smaller. However above a diameter of about 0.4mm, the system changes and single numbers are used, which increase in size as the suture diameter gets larger.

20. B **The forceps used for laying out an instrument trolley are Cheatle forceps**

Rampley's forceps are used to apply skin preparation solutions, and Rochester-Pean and Crile's forceps are both types of artery forceps.

21. A **A laparotomy incision made parallel to, but to one side of, the linea alba can be described as paramedian**

Paracostal incisions are made parallel to the costal arch at the cranial end of the abdomen.

Sublumbar incisions are made ventral to the wing of the ilium (as for a cat spay), and midline incisions are made through the linea alba in the ventral midline of the patient. This last approach is the most common laparotomy incision used.

18 Fluid therapy and shock

1. B **A small water-soluble particle which carries one or more positive charges is called a cation**

An anion is the same, but negatively charged, and the term ion is a more general word which is used to denote any charged particle in solution. Electrolytes are substances that dissociate to form ions when dissolved in water.

2. D **The main intracellular anions are phosphate and protein**

Protein might not immediately seem to be an anion, but in solution, proteins have a tendency to lose hydrogen ions, and therefore become negatively charged.

Remember that sodium and chloride are always found together, and sodium is the main extracellular cation, so chloride too will be extracellular.

Finally, sodium and calcium are positively charged ions which makes them cations. These are found mainly in the extracellular fluids.

3. B **Normally a healthy animal will generate about 10% of its daily water requirement through metabolic processes**

This is often referred to as metabolic water.

4. B **A urine specific gravity measurement of 1.010 is within the isosthenuric range**

Isosthenuria refers to urine which has neither been concentrated or diluted as it has passed through the renal tubule, and is therefore the same concentration as a filtrate of plasma. The range of SGs within this bracket are 1.008 – 1.015.

5. C   **The estimated fluid deficit for this dog is 1000 ml**

To calculate a fluid deficit based on a PCV reading the animal's original PCV should be known. However, this is rarely the case, and usually an estimate of 45% is used.

To calculate the deficit the following is used – that for every 1% increase in PCV, 10ml/kg fluid has been lost.

This dog has a PCV increase of $(50 - 45) = 5\%$

Therefore the volume required $= 5 \times 10$ ml/kg $\times 20$ kg
$= 1000$ ml

6. A   **Metabolic acidosis could be caused by chronic renal failure**

In chronic renal failure the animal loses considerable amounts of bicarbonate in the urine, and therefore becomes acidotic.

With prepyloric vomiting, the main electrolytes lost are hydrogen and chloride ions from the hydrochloric acid in the stomach. This patient would become alkalotic.

Conditions involving the respiratory tract would not be referred to as metabolic conditions, but would be described as respiratory alkalosis (for example due to hyperventilation) or respiratory acidosis (as could be caused by lung damage).

7. C   **An over-the-needle catheter should be replaced every 48 hours**

If left in place longer than this, it would predispose to the development of thrombophlebitis. Changing the catheter more frequently than this would damage the vein unnecessarily.

8. D   **Intraosseous administration would be the most suitable route for fluid therapy for a severely dehydrated puppy**

This route provides direct access to the medullary cavity and therefore to the bone marrow. Blood cells produced in the marrow enter the circulation via blood vessels leaving the centre of the bone, so fluids administered to this site are also able to enter the circulation directly.

Subcutaneous, intraperitoneal and rectal administration are

not suitable for severely dehydrated animals as the rate of uptake of the fluids is too slow to be beneficial.

9. C   Acid citrate dextrose is the anticoagulant generally used when collecting blood for a blood transfusion

Two anticoagulants are available specifically for blood transfusions – acid citrate dextrose (ACD) and citrate phosphate dextrose (CPD). However heparin or EDTA may be used in an emergency, though these are more routinely used for blood analysis in the laboratory. Fluoride-oxalate is used if glucose estimations are required, and sodium citrate may be used if coagulation studies are to be carried out.

10. B   Dextran solutions are hypertonic

These contain high molecular weight dextran molecules, and are one of the two types of colloid preparation available.

Gelatins such as Haemaccel® and Gelofusin® are both isotonic solutions, as are the other crystalloid solutions listed.

11. B   It is unsafe to add sodium bicarbonate to Hartmann's or Ringer's solution since it reacts with calcium to form a solid precipitate

Calcium reacts with sodium bicarbonate to form calcium carbonate which is insoluble in water (and is the main component of chalk!).

The other statements are all untrue.

12. D   An animal which was becoming overhydrated would not show oliguria

Oliguria is reduced urinary output. Providing that the urinary system was still functioning normally, then the animal would actually show an increased urine output.

The other signs all relate to overhydration – the nasal discharge and respiratory distress would be due to pulmonary oedema, and chemosis (bulging of the conjunctiva) can be due to conjunctival oedema.

13. D   Hypertension is not normally seen in shock

Raised blood pressure would not be seen – most shocked animals are hypotensive, either due to fluid loss, or maldistribution of fluids.

14. B   0.18% saline + 4% dextrose would be the most appropriate fluid to use for maintenance requirements

The crystalloids all have specific uses, and although this is not always adhered to in practice, it is important that veterinary nurses have an understanding of which product should be used when.

Hartmann's is very useful for post-gastric vomiting and diarrhoea. Ringer's solution does not contain lactate, and is therefore used for vomiting losses. 5% dextrose is used in primary water deficits and hypoglycaemia.

15. B   The correct drip rate is 1 drop per second

First, calculate the volume to be given in 6 hours:

2880 ÷ 2 = 1440 ml in 6 hours

The hourly and minute rate are then calculated:

1440 ÷ 6 = 240 ml in 1 hour

240 ÷ 60 = 4 ml in 1 minute

Now the drip factor is incorporated, remembering that 1 ml = 15 drops:

4 x 15 = 60 drops in 1 minute

Finally the drops per second are worked out:

60 ÷ 60 = 1 drop per second

19 Anaesthesia and analgesia

1. C   It is not true that older animals are always at greater risk than young patients

Risk varies more with the patient's condition than with actual chronological age. Therefore an old fit Labrador may pose far fewer problems under anaesthetic than a small kitten.

Liver disease usually results in a delay in metabolism of anaesthetic agents, so the animal remains unconscious for longer.

Animals treated for epilepsy are usually given phenobarbitone, and this induces an increase in liver enzymes. This therefore has the opposite effect to liver disease – the anaesthetic agents may be metabolised more quickly than usual.

Patients with renal disease should certainly be supported with fluid therapy since they are more prone to renal ischaemia due to reduced blood flow, and consequent acute renal failure.

2. A   Xylazine is an alpha-2 agonist

Drugs described as alpha-2 agonists stimulate alpha-2 adrenoreceptors in the central nervous system which inhibit the release of noradrenaline. The two used in general practice are xylazine, as mentioned above, and medetomidine.

Atipamezole is an alpha-2 antagonist, and this reverses the effect of medetomidine.

Diazepam is a benzodiazepine. This group also includes midazolam and both these drugs are useful tranquillisers in debilitated patients.

Acepromazine is a phenothiazine, and is widely used as a premedicant.

3. B   The only drug listed that has no analgesic effect is acepromazine

All the others can be used as analgesics, though each works at a different site and in a different way.

4. D   Buprenorphine has the longest duration of action (6-8 hours)

Pethidine is the shortest acting drug, with a duration of 1-2 hours. Morphine and butorphanol both last 3-4 hours.

5. D   Non-steroidal anti-inflammatories may cause gastric irritation

The other drugs are not known to cause this side effect, though each group may cause other problems.

6. C   The addition of adrenaline to local anaesthetic preparations increases the duration of the nerve block

This is achieved by causing local vasoconstriction, and therefore reducing the rate of anaesthetic absorption and removal by the bloodstream.

7. B   The concentration of a 5% solution in mg/ml is 50 mg/ml

The definition of a % solution is 5g in 100ml.

This is the same as 5000mg in 100ml.

This is the same as 50mg in 1 ml or 50 mg/ml.

(Alternatively, simply remember that to convert from % to mg/ml you always need to multiply by 10.)

8. C   A perineural block is defined as injection of local anaesthetic in the proximity of an identifiable nerve

This type of technique is gaining in popularity since perineural blocks can be used to provide post-operative analgesia. For example, intercostal nerves may be specifically blocked after a thoracotomy to provide pain relief. The technique is also used diagnostically in equine practice to identify the location of pain in a horse that is lame.

Surface blocks are achieved simply by applying the anaesthetic topically. Epidural blocks are given into the epidural space, just outside the meninges of the spinal cord. This blocks the spinal nerves as they emerge from the spinal cord.

IVRA stands for intravenous regional anaesthesia. It is achieved with the use of a tourniquet, and intravenous injection of the local anaesthetic distal to the tourniquet. The whole area distal to the tourniquet will be desensitised until the tourniquet is removed.

9. A   Thiopentone, if injected perivascularly, may cause tissue necrosis

Thiopentone is very alkaline (pH 10.5) and therefore can cause severe problems if high concentrations are used.

10. B   Saffan is a steroid

More accurately it is in fact a mixture of two steroids (alphaxalone and alphadolone) in an oil base.

The barbiturates include thiopentone. Ketamine is a dissociative anaesthetic and propofol is a phenol.

11. A   The MAC number provides information about the potency of the drug

MAC stands for Minimum Alveolar Concentration and is the alveolar concentration of the drug that prevents a response to a given surgical stimulus in 50% of animals.

Agents with high MAC numbers are therefore less potent, since a higher concentration of drug is required to achieve the same effect as a drug with a lower MAC number.

12. B   Sevoflurane degrades in the presence of soda-lime

Sevoflurane is a relatively new product that is now being

used in some surgeries in the UK. It is a good anaesthetic, but relatively unstable, and degrades in the presence of soda-lime to produce metabolites which have been shown to be toxic to rats. However, the manufacturers do not believe this to be the case with other species.

13. C   The least potent inhalation agent is nitrous oxide

Nitrous oxide has a MAC number of 188-220, which means that the alveoli would need to be more than 100% filled with nitrous in order to stop an animal feeling and reacting to a stimulus. It cannot therefore be used as an anaesthetic agent on its own, though it is useful in reducing the amount of other agent needed.

Animals anaesthetised with sevoflurane show rapid induction and recovery. It is less potent than isoflurane, which is now widely used in small animal practice.

Methoxyflurane is the most potent inhalation agent, but induction and recovery are relatively slow. It is not commonly seen in general practice though it provides good analgesia.

14. B   It is untrue that passive scavenging requires the use of a fan

Passive scavenging is achieved either by a short piece of tubing leading to the outside, or to a canister containing activated charcoal.

Active scavenge methods require the use of fans.

The other statements about scavenging are true.

15. B   The normal ratio of nitrous oxide to oxygen in inhalation anaesthesia is 2:1

A minimum level of oxygen must always be provided since nitrous oxide binds quite effectively with haemoglobin and therefore competes with any available oxygen.

16. D   The Magill circuit is not suitable for prolonged IPPV

The other circuits are all good for performing IPPV if required.

17. C   200 ml/kg/min may be used as an estimate of an animal's minute volume in order to calculate the fresh gas flow rate

This allows for both the number of breaths per minute and the tidal volume of the animal.

18. A   The circuit factor for a Lack circuit is 1 – 1.5

This is the factor that should be used and multiplied by the minute volume in order to calculate the fresh gas flow rate.

19. D   Size E cylinders are usually used for small portable anaesthetic machines

Size E cylinders contain 680 litres of oxygen. Size F cylinders may also be used, and these contain 1340 litres.

Larger practices use piped gases, and these are supplied by size G or J cylinders.

20. B   The gas contained in grey cylinders is carbon dioxide

Oxygen is always supplied in black cylinders with a white neck.

Blue cylinders contain nitrous oxide, and cyclopropane (rarely used now) was delivered in orange cylinders.

21. A   The statement that gallamine is the most commonly used neuro-muscular blocker is untrue

Gallamine is relatively unpopular due to tachycardia and hypertension after its use. Succinyl choline, vecuronium and atracurium are probably the most widely used agents.

22. D   Edrophonium can be used to antagonise neuro-muscular blockade

Naloxone (Narcan) is the drug used in humans to counteract the effect of the opiate component of Immobilon, whereas diprenorphine is the active component of Revivon, the reversal agent for Immobilon for use in small animals.

Atipamezole (Antisedan) reverses medetomidine (Domitor).

23. A   **Stage I is the stage of voluntary excitement**

The four stages of anaesthesia are less applicable now than in the past since the categories are based on ether anaesthesia in humans. However they are still frequently referred to.

Stage II is involuntary excitement. Stage III is surgical anaesthesia, and Stage IV is overdosage.

24. C   **Bright pink mucous membranes might suggest hypercapnia**

Pink mucous membranes are desirable since this would show good perfusion, but if they become bright pink this could indicate too much carbon dioxide in the system.

25. A   **Thiopentone sodium is the drug that is metabolised the slowest**

Both thiopentone and methohexitone are barbiturates, but methohexitone is metabolised far more quickly, which makes it a useful barbiturate to use in lean dogs.

Propofol (Rapinovet) is very rapidly metabolised, as is alphaxalone and alphadolone (Saffan).

26. A   **The correct description is that the Magill consists of a single piece of tubing with the valve close to the animal and the reservoir bag close to the anaesthetic machine**

27. D   **Vaporisers should not be filled at the start of an operating session**

Vaporisers should be filled at the end of the working day, ensuring that the environment is well ventilated.

All the other statements are recommendations made by the Health and Safety Executive in respect of the use of anaesthetics in practice.

28. C   **It is true that neonates should be starved for no longer than 2-3 hours**

Many of the body systems are not yet fully developed in the

neonate, and care must be taken to ensure that support is given whilst under anaesthesia.

Oxygen consumption in a neonate is actually 2-3 times higher than in the adult, hypotension is quite likely to occur unless care is taken, and drug dosages will need to be reduced, not increased, to account for the immaturity of the animal.

29. B Surgery on the eye may lead to a reflex slowing of the heart rate

If pressure is placed on the eye this may result in a reflex stimulation of the vagus nerve which causes the heart rate to slow. The reflex is called the oculo-vagal reflex.

Surgery on the lateral aspect of the neck close to the jugular groove may also cause a vagal response since the vagus runs close to this site. However thyroid surgery should not impinge on the vagus which lies more laterally.

30. D Dobutamine may be used in cases of hypotension

Dobutamine can be used to deal with cases of emergency hypotension. It is most effective if given in conjunction with intravenous fluids, in which case the simplest access route is via the intravenous line. It is a positive inotrope, and acts to increase the force of cardiac contractions.

Atropine is indicated in cardiac arrest or vagal bradycardias.

Lignocaine is used in cases of ventricular tachycardia and bicarbonate is used for cases of acidosis.

20 Diagnostic imaging

1. D   **It is true that all waves on the electromagnetic spectrum travel at the same speed**

Wavelength is inversely proportional to the frequency, thus waves with high frequencies (such as X-rays) have very short wavelengths.

X-rays are one of several ionising radiations which include γ-rays, and α and β-particles. X-rays and γ-rays are part of the electromagnetic spectrum, whereas α and β-particles are not.

2. B   **The function of the aluminium filter across the window of the X-ray tube head is to absorb 'soft' or low-powered X-rays**

The other statements are untrue.

3. C   **The function of the oil bath is to act as a heat sink, for the heat generated at the target of the tube head**

4. D   **It is untrue that the mA control alters the potential difference between the cathode and the anode of the X-ray tube head**

The mA control determines the electrical current passing through the tungsten filament. If this is increased the heating of the filament increases and more electrons are produced, which means that more X-rays are generated.

It is the kV control that determines the potential difference between the cathode and anode of the tube head. This affects the speed of the electrons as they travel across the tube head and the subsequent energy of the emerging X-rays. The kV is only applied for a short time, which is determined by the timer control.

5. B **An operator should be at least 2 metres away from the primary beam when making an exposure**

For machines which have the exposure button on a lead, this means that the lead should be at least 2 metres in length. More modern or more powerful machines may have a separate control panel which is away from the tube head – either behind a lead screen or outside the X-ray room itself.

6. A **If a radiograph was taken and the kV was too high, all tissues would be overpenetrated and the whole radiograph would be dark**

If the kV was too low, then the subject would be underpenetrated, and the image would appear pale with a black background.

If the image was pale with a pale background, this is most likely to be due to underdevelopment, especially if the film was developed manually.

7. D **The correct formula to adjust the mAs when changing the focal-film distance is:**

$$\text{New mAs} = \text{Old mAs} \times \frac{\text{New distance}^2}{\text{Old distance}^2}$$

8. B **The use of a grid does not reduce the amount of scattered radiation produced**

Grids are designed to prevent scatter reaching the film and affecting the quality of the image. They require the use of greater exposure factors which actually increases the amount of scatter produced.

The other methods listed all have the effect of reducing scatter.

9. B **The focused grid is the most effective at avoiding grid cut off**

The parallel grid is the cheapest of the grids, but since the primary beam diverges this suffers from so called grid cut off at the edges of the plate.

Focused grids have tapered slats so that the divergent beam

is still able to pass through these and reach the film.

Pseudo-focused grids have parallel slats that get progressively shorter towards the edge of the grid. This is an improvement on the parallel grid, but still not as good as the focused grid.

Crossed grids have the slats running in both directions across the plate. These can be either parallel or focused.

10. C   It is the emulsion that contains the X-ray sensitive grains of silver bromide

The supercoat is a protective layer which lies directly over the surface of the emulsion. The subbing layer is a sticky material required to attach the emulsion to the polyester base beneath.

11. D   Non-screen film requires the highest exposures

Screen film is used in conjunction with a cassette and intensifying screens. The screens convert X-rays into light which adds to the direct effect of X-rays on the film. Fast film has large silver bromide grains and requires the lowest exposures, but this is at the expense of the crispness of the image. At the other end of the spectrum, non-screen film requires high exposures, but gives very good fine detail.

Mammography film is single-sided film, used with a cassette, so it uses lower exposures than non-screen film, but still requires about five times the exposure levels of standard double-sided film.

12. A   The active chemical in the developer is phenidone hydroquinone

Ammonium thiosulphate and sodium thiosulphate are both chemicals used in fixer solutions. Silver halide is an alternative way of describing the silver bromide grains in the emulsion in the film.

13. C   For manual processing the temperature of the developer tank is usually kept at 20°C

In an automatic processor developing temperatures are much higher, usually in the region of 28°C.

14. A   The somatic effects of X-rays are changes in tissues exposed to radiation, such as damage to the intestinal wall, leading to vomiting and dehydration

Other somatic effects include damage to the developing foetus, baldness and cataract formation.

The other effects described are carcinogenic and genetic effects rather than somatic.

15. B   The minimum thickness of lead equivalence required for a lead apron is 0.25 mm

This varies for differing types of clothing. Gloves and sleeves should be at least 0.35 mm lead equivalent.

Lead clothing does not provide protection against the primary beam; it is designed to simply protect the wearer against scatter, and so no part of any person, even when covered in lead clothing, should ever be placed in the primary beam.

16. D   It is untrue that barium sulphate can be used in the respiratory tract to highlight the trachea and bronchi

Barium may cause pneumonia if aspirated, and therefore should never be used in the respiratory tract. It should also not be used in cases of suspect perforation, since if it leaks into the thoracic or abdominal cavities it can lead to the development of granulomas or adhesions.

17. B   The technique used to highlight the ureters is intravenous urography (IVU)

There are several techniques used to show up the urinary system. IVU techniques mean that the contrast medium is given intravenously, and then passes through the kidneys as the blood is filtered. The positive medium can be traced through the ureters to the bladder.

The other techniques all rely on the placement of a urinary catheter, and the administration of the contrast media either directly into the bladder or more caudally into the urethra. The contrast medium does not flow back into the ureters using these techniques.

18. C   Ultrasound waves are produced due to the piezo-electric effect

The photo-electric effect and Compton effect both result from the interaction of X-rays with matter. Thermionic emission describes the way in which electrons are generated by passing an electric current through the tungsten filament in the tube head.

19. A   A screening scheme using ultrasonography has been set up for polycystic kidney disease in cats

The Feline Advisory Bureau set up this scheme in November 2000 to attempt to reduce the incidence of the disease in certain breeds of cat such as the Persian and Exotic Shorthair.

20. C   Scintigraphy relies on the use of radioactive substances injected into the patient and a gamma camera

This is mainly used in horses, but more recently is also being used in cats to image the thyroid gland in cases of hyperthyroidism.

21. C   Unexposed silver halide is removed from the film during fixing

During development, exposed silver halide is converted into solid silver, and then during fixing the film is cleared of the remaining unchanged silver bromide.

22. B   The X-ray beam should be centred level with the caudal border of the scapula, midway between the dorsal and ventral skin surfaces for a radiograph of the lateral thorax

23. A   **The settings that could be used are 70kV, 20 mA and 0.5 seconds**

In order to be able to work this out, you need to remember the rule of thumb that states:

If you increase the kV by 10, you may halve the mAs.

It also works in reverse. Thus if you decrease the kV by 10, you have to double the mAs.

So in this instance, the original mAs $= 10 \times 0.5 = 5$ mAs

The new mAs, using a kV of 70,
is now double the original: $= 5 \times 2 = 10$ mAs

Therefore to find the answer, simply check the answers given to see which one has a mAs of 10, with 70 kV. There is just one possibility – answer A.

24. C   **Non-screen film should be left in the developer for 5 minutes when manual processing at standard temperatures**

Normal film takes 4 minutes in the developer, but because the emulsion of non-screen film is thicker it takes slightly longer for the chemicals to penetrate fully.

Printed and bound by CPI Group (UK) Ltd, Croydon, CR0 4YY

03/10/2024

01040848-0004